Principles of Specialty Nursing

Under the Auspices of the European
Specialist Nurses Organisations (ESNO)

Series Editor
Ber Oomen, Executive Director,
European Specialist Nurses Organisation,
Arnhem, The Netherlands

The role of the specialist nurse in Europe is still not clearly defined. Despite the fact that there have been formal training programs – e.g. for nurse anaesthetists, operating room nurses, intensive care and mental health nurses – for years now, the practices, status, duration and content of training can vary greatly from country to country. Some other specialist roles, e.g. for Diabetes, Dialysis, Urology and Oncology, have successfully been established in Europe with the help of professional transnational collaborations.

Moreover, advances in medical technologies and more sophisticated treatment will not only require specialist nurses in order to ensure quality and safety of care, but will also call upon them to assume new roles in their professional field to compensate for physician shortages. Most of the available literature on specialty nursing practice currently comes from the USA, Canada, and Australia, and accordingly reflects evidence-based nursing in these countries.

Therefore, there is a need to establish European evidence-based practice on the basis of different clinical experiences. This series, which encompasses textbooks for each specialty, shapes evidence-based practice in Europe, while also integrating lessons learned from other continents. Moreover, it contributes to clarifying the status of the specialist nurse as an advanced practice nurse.

Each volume is dedicated to a specialty such as Mental health and Pyschiatry, firstly published, but also Oncology, Kidney Care, Prevention Control, Vaccination etc. and for most of them, textbooks are supported by ESNO member societies.

Ber Oomen • Silvana Gastaldi
Editors

Principles of Nursing Infection Prevention Control

Introduction and global context of Infection Prevention and Control (Volume 1)

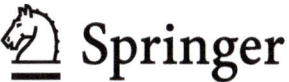 Springer

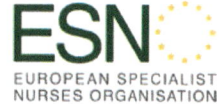

Editors
Ber Oomen
European Specialist Nurses
Organisation (ESNO)
Arnhem, The Netherlands

Silvana Gastaldi
Independent Researcher
Mazzano, Italy

ISSN 2366-875X   ISSN 2366-8768   (electronic)
Principles of Specialty Nursing
ISBN 978-3-031-84468-3   ISBN 978-3-031-84469-0   (eBook)
https://doi.org/10.1007/978-3-031-84469-0

This Springer imprint is published by the registered company Springer Nature Switzerland AG
The registered company address is: Gewerbestrasse 11, 6330 Cham, Switzerland

If disposing of this product, please recycle the paper.

Foreword

The recent pandemic has highlighted more than ever the personal, financial and ethical importance of preventing infection. Public and professional awareness of the impact of respiratory infections continues to dominate public debate like never before. Driven increasingly by social media beyond the traditional boundaries of health and care settings the effect of infection on schools, workplaces and enclosed indoor spaces remains. Likewise current outbreaks and spread of rare or re-emerging infections continue to capture the media and public imagination. Zoonotic infections such as Mpox, Marberg, Oropouche, highly pathogenic avian influenza and *M. tuberculosis* remind us of human vulnerability to the effects of climatic change and human migration despite the arsenal of medicines and vaccines available to combat disease. Closer to home antibiotic resistance continues as a "silent pandemic" threatening our ability to deliver modern healthcare and the ever-increasing technically feasible procedures to save and extend life.

At the centre of this reality lies the nursing profession. As advocates for patient and public safety the prevention of infection is central to our role and ethical codes of conduct. Whilst the focus historically is on the technical aspects of process or technique, for example, insertion of invasive devices, hand hygiene or decontamination, this post-pandemic era offers opportunities to reshape and redesign infection prevention beyond the procedural and historical limits of healthcare. The need to traverse invisible boundaries dictated so often by funding streams between physical and mental health, prevention and treatment, community and hospital-based care is now critical as the effects of climate change become embedded and escalate.

This book leads the readers through the evolution of infection prevention to the current day and beyond with a clear focus on how, as a practical specialism, global perspectives and learning across different specialties, scientific disciplines or care settings offer unique opportunities. The diversity of authors reflects a global focus which is both contemporary and welcome. I commend the authors for their collaborative and insightful approach to re-focus infection prevention and control through critical thinking and reflection as nurses working in one of the most interesting, complex and challenging specialties of our time.

Royal College of Nursing   Rose Gallagher
London, UK

In Memoriam: Bjørg Marit Andersen

It is with great sadness that we announce the passing of Bjørg Marit Andersen on July 8, 2024, at the age of 82. A pioneering expert in infection prevention, her profound impact on nursing and care for the elderly will resonate for years. Bjørg was a passionate advocate for vulnerable populations, particularly those in nursing homes. Her commitment to infection prevention was evident in her extensive research and publications, as well as her fearless approach to addressing critical healthcare issues.

Bjørg's contributions to the field were significant, with her work published at Springer. Her notable work, "Prevention and Control of Infections in Hospitals: Practice and Theory," provides vital information on infection control procedures. In "Patient Protection Is Patient Safety," she emphasizes the importance of effective measures for patient safety. Her chapter "Hospital Infections: Surveillance" details methods for preventing hospital-acquired infections. We also miss her contributions to the ESNO series, where she elaborated on the history of nurses in infection prevention.

Her publications were invaluable resources for healthcare professionals and students, showcasing her dedication to advancing knowledge and best practices. Bjørg's unique blend of expertise and compassion always prioritized the dignity of those she protected. She inspired countless healthcare professionals to adopt best practices and advocate for necessary reforms, leaving a legacy that will inspire future generations to prioritize the health of the elderly.

As we reflect on her remarkable life, we honor Bjørg Marit Andersen not just as a leader in infection prevention but as a champion for those who often had no voice. Her courage and dedication will be profoundly missed, but her impact will forever endure in the hearts of those she inspired.

Ber Oomen
Silvana Gastaldi
Nathalie Lhorset-Poulain

Preface

Infection prevention and control (IPC) is a critical element in safeguarding public health, where practitioners are at the frontline of patient care. As the world faces an ever-evolving landscape of infectious threats—from hospital-acquired infections to global pandemics—the need for comprehensive, evidence-based strategies in IPC has never been more urgent. *Principles of Nursing Infection Prevention Control* seeks to address these challenges by offering a detailed exploration of infection prevention within diverse contexts, combining historical insights with cutting-edge practices and global perspectives.

This two-volume work has been meticulously curated to serve as both a foundational text for those new to the field and a valuable resource for experienced professionals seeking to refine their practice. Volume 1 introduces readers to the global context of infection prevention, highlighting the essential role nurses play in maintaining patient safety, while also examining the historical and legislative frameworks that shape IPC today. Volume 2 delves into the practical applications of IPC across a variety of environments, emphasizing preparedness and adaptability in diverse healthcare settings.

By fostering an understanding of the fundamental principles of infection control and encouraging a multidisciplinary approach, this book aims to equip healthcare professionals with the tools needed to mitigate infection risks and promote patient safety across all levels of care. We hope this work serves as a catalyst for ongoing education, research, and innovation in this critical field.

Independent Researcher, Mazzano, Italy   Silvana Gastaldi
Arnhem, The Netherlands   Ber Oomen

Acknowledgments

This book on nurses and infection prevention would not have been possible without the contributions of many individuals and organizations. First, we extend our deepest gratitude to the authors who generously shared their expertise, insights, and experience. Each chapter reflects the dedication of professionals committed to advancing the field of infection prevention in healthcare. Their knowledge and passion have made this book a valuable resource for both current and future healthcare practitioners.

We are also deeply thankful to the experts we consulted throughout the development of this book. Their guidance, feedback, and specialized knowledge have significantly enhanced the quality of the work. Their contributions ensured that the content aligns with the latest trends, best practices, and innovations in infection prevention, making the book not only relevant but impactful for the broader healthcare community.

A special thanks goes to the Springer editorial team, whose support and professionalism were instrumental in the successful publication of this work. We are proud to be part of the Springer series under the European Specialist Nurses Organization (ESNO), and we appreciate the opportunity to contribute to this important body of knowledge. The Springer team's expertise in producing high-quality academic content has been invaluable, and we are grateful for their partnership throughout the process.

Our sincere thanks also go to Nathalie L'horset-Poulain and the program lead for their dedication and leadership in making this project possible. Their vision and commitment to strengthening the role of specialist nurses in infection prevention have been inspiring, and we are deeply appreciative of their tireless support and contributions.

To our friends and families, we owe a special debt of gratitude for their patience, understanding, and encouragement throughout the entire process. Their unwavering support provided us with the strength and motivation needed to see this project through to completion, even during the most challenging moments.

Finally, we wish to thank the wider specialist nursing community, including the members of ESNO and our many associates. Your dedication to improving healthcare through infection prevention is inspiring, and this book stands as a reflection of your hard work and commitment. We are honored to be part of such a passionate and forward-thinking group of professionals.

To everyone involved in this journey, thank you for your invaluable contributions. We look forward to continuing this work together and are excited to begin work on Volume 2.

Silvana Gastaldi
Ber Oomen

Contents

About the Editors

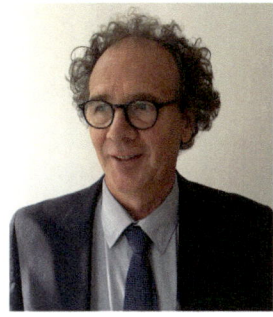

Ber Oomen serves as the Executive Director of the European Specialist Nurses Organization (ESNO), where he leads efforts to promote the role of specialist and advanced nurses across Europe. His work focuses on empowering nurses by enhancing their professional development and well-being. A champion of nurse leadership, he is actively involved in various initiatives, including leading focus groups on vaccination. Ber participates in numerous European projects aimed at strengthening nursing roles in healthcare systems, while also contributing to national initiatives in the Netherlands. His leadership highlights the crucial role of nurses in specialized fields, advancing their impact on patient care, public health, and professional autonomy.

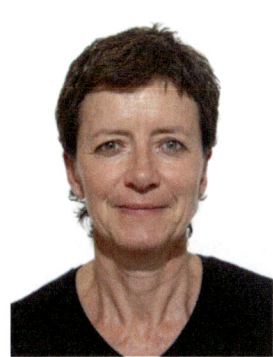

Silvana Gastaldi Beginning with master's degrees in biology and nursing, her career has spanned multiple domains. She has worked as a consultant, supporting organizations in achieving ISO 9001, ISO 14000, and Joint Commission International (JCI) certifications. After transitioning to the Italian's National Health Service (NHS), she practiced as a nurse across various departments while simultaneously teaching in support of hospital certification programs. Her humanitarian involvement began in 2014, leading to diverse roles with international organizations in emergency response, outbreak management, and healthcare training. Her academic path continued with advanced studies in nursing management and coordination, disaster medicine, and the prevention of healthcare-associated infections, alongside a research contract with the University of Verona focusing on SARS-CoV-2, infection prevention and control (IPC), and antimicrobial resistance (AMR).

She has collaborated with the World Health Organization (WHO) and national health authorities on IPC program development and is currently engaged in scientific work on IPC with the Italian National Institute of Health (Istituto Superiore di Sanità, ISS) and humanitarian organizations.

Preambles: Toward the Future

Joséphine Declaye

1.1 Introduction

Infection prevention and control (IPC) has become a cornerstone of modern health-care, as we have entered an era marked by unprecedented challenges. Emerging infectious diseases, the rapid rise of antimicrobial resistance (AMR), and global pandemics, such as COVID-19, have exposed vulnerabilities within healthcare systems. These crises have also highlighted the critical role of nurses and healthcare professionals in safeguarding public health.

Today's nurses play a multifaceted role that goes far beyond the basics of infection control. Equipped with advanced diagnostic tools and educated in antimicrobial stewardship, they are pivotal in public health education, patient care, and the integration of cutting-edge technologies into routine practice. Nurses must actively engage in interprofessional collaboration. They will lead the development of sustainable care system, long-term infection prevention strategies with activities such as those described above. Identifying early signs of infection, educating patients on the proper use of their treatments, promoting hand hygiene, and ensuring access to clean water. Their leadership will be guided by wise decision-making, thoughtfully balancing available options to benefit individuals, healthcare systems, and society as a whole.

More research is needed to guide the development of novel interventions to address crucial knowledge gaps in pathogen- and infection-specific burdens [1].

As we move toward 2030 and beyond, the clinical pipeline for new antibiotics is drying. The world risks sliding back into a preantibiotic era. This crisis could reverse decades of medical progress. The rise of antimicrobial resistance (AMR) poses a significant threat. With common antibiotics becoming less effective, routine procedures such

J. Declaye (✉)
Simulation Center, Department of Public Health, University of Liège, Liège, Belgium

SIZ Nursing, Society of Intensive Care Nurses, Brussels, Belgium

© The Author(s), under exclusive license to Springer Nature Switzerland AG 2025
B. Oomen, S. Gastaldi (eds.), *Principles of Nursing Infection Prevention Control*,
Principles of Specialty Nursing, https://doi.org/10.1007/978-3-031-84469-0_1

as surgeries, cancer treatments, and organ transplants may once again carry life-threatening risks owing to uncontrollable infections. As seen during the COVID-19 pandemic, global healthcare systems must urgently adapt to prevent further setbacks [2].

When an individual dies from sepsis, the probability that the organism causing infection is drug resistant was 25% higher in 2019 than in 1990/ [3].

In 2019, AMR was responsible for 1.3 million deaths worldwide, disproportionately affecting low- and middle-income countries. Without urgent action, this figure will only rise. The UN General Assembly High-Level Meeting on AMR in 2024 set clear targets, including reducing deaths associated with bacterial AMR by 10% by 2030. The political declaration [4] adopted during this meeting reflects the global recognition of this threat, but there is still much work to be done, especially in terms of funding and innovation.

1.2   Monitoring

One of the key challenges facing the future of IPC is the need for real-time monitoring systems to detect and manage infections and monitor therapies, particularly those caused by resistant organisms. Today's nurses are increasingly expected to utilize advanced digital surveillance tools that track infection patterns, monitor antimicrobial use, and detect the spread of resistant organisms in real time. These systems increase the ability of nurses to make data-driven decisions, allowing for faster identification of infection outbreaks and more accurate antimicrobial stewardship. As advocates for patient safety, nurses must not only use these tools effectively but also ensure that they are fully integrated into clinical workflows.

The next generation of nurses must view themselves not only as care providers but also as data interpreters, using digital health tools to increase patient safety and infection control practices. By contributing to the design and improvement of these systems, nurses can ensure that real-time monitoring becomes a cornerstone of future IPC efforts. Being part of the solution is key.

One of the most promising innovations in infection control is the use of rapid diagnostic tools and point-of-care (POC) testing, which provide immediate information about the type of infection and its antimicrobial resistance profile. These tools allow nurses to act swiftly and precisely, ensuring that infections are treated with the appropriate medications—reducing the unnecessary use of antibiotics and limiting the spread of resistant bacteria.

Mastering point-of-care (POC) testing is a critical skill for the next generation of nurses. These rapid tests allow for the differentiation between bacterial and viral infections, ensuring that antibiotics are only prescribed when absolutely necessary, thus reducing their overuse. However, the true challenge lies in integrating these technologies into routine nursing practice without sacrificing patient-centered care. Nurses need to balance the use of new technologies with clinical judgment, considering each patient's unique circumstances.

In addition to managing individual cases, nurses play a key role in recognizing outbreaks and clusters of infections. Early identification of patterns, whether in a hospital setting or community healthcare, will allow swift action to contain infections before they spread. By leveraging real-time data from POC testing and digital infection monitoring tools, nurses can detect unusual spikes in infection rates and work with interdisciplinary teams to investigate potential outbreaks or clusters.

Recognizing clusters is vital not only for curbing the unnecessary use of antibiotics but also for limiting the spread of resistant bacteria. When clusters are caught early, appropriate containment measures can be implemented, and the use of antibiotics can be more targeted, preventing broader misuse that fuels antimicrobial resistance. For nurses, staying vigilant in these patterns and combining technological tools with observation will be key to maintaining infection control in the long run.

The deployment of rapid diagnostic tests in low-resource settings will present an opportunity for nurses to extend the reach of effective infection control beyond hospitals and into the broader community.

1.3   Interprofessional Collaboration

Antimicrobial resistance (AMR) represents one of the most significant threats to global health in the twenty-first century. Nurses are not only central to delivering care but also play a crucial role in ensuring that antimicrobials are used appropriately. This is particularly true in the case of antibiotics, which, if overused or misused, can lead to the development of drug-resistant bacteria [3].

One of the major challenges in modern healthcare is collaboration to address complex issues such as infection control and AMR. Nurses, as frontline healthcare workers, must work closely with physicians, pharmacists, microbiologists, and public health officials to ensure a coordinated and effective response to infections.

Programs aimed at preparing nurses for the future must therefore adopt teaching strategies and methods that allow nurses to develop the interprofessional skills necessary to practice collaboratively. This includes training in communication, teamwork, and leadership—skills that enable nurses to take active roles in multidisciplinary teams. Collaborative practice ensures that patient care is holistic, drawing on the expertise of multiple disciplines to provide the most effective infection prevention strategies.

Nurses must be empowered not only to implement infection control measures but also to lead initiatives in healthcare settings, advocating for best practices and ensuring that all team members are aligned with evidence-based guidelines. Nurses should view themselves as collaborative leaders who can bring together various healthcare professionals to address infections, particularly in the context of increasing AMR. Stewardship programs are effective in achieving this goal.

1.4   Antimicrobial Stewardship

Nurses are in a unique position to influence patient behaviors regarding antibiotic use. Through education and direct communication on infection risks and preventive measures, nurses can ensure that patients understand the importance of completing prescribed antibiotic courses and the dangers of self-medication. In antimicrobial stewardship programs, nurses collaborate with pharmacists, physicians, and microbiologists to ensure that antimicrobial therapies are based on accurate diagnostic criteria. Nurses play a crucial role in patient education, explaining the importance of adhering to prescribed treatments and the risks of antibiotic misuse. Furthermore, nurses actively participate in auditing antimicrobial usage, ensuring compliance with stewardship protocols, and advocating the reduction of unnecessary prescriptions [5, 6].

Nurses face the challenge of integrating stewardship principles into everyday practice. This means understanding the local and global patterns of AMR, being proactive in infection prevention, and promoting the use of vaccines and other preventive measures to reduce the need for antimicrobial agents. Nurses must also be prepared to challenge inappropriate antibiotic use and advocate for policies that support responsible antimicrobial prescribing practices in their institutions.

By understanding the global threat of AMR and being equipped with the latest knowledge, nurses can advocate for sustainable antibiotic use and ensure that appropriate treatments are administered. This is particularly crucial in areas where antibiotic misuse is rampant due to a lack of education or access to healthcare [5].

1.5   Reducing the Need for Antibiotics

One of the most promising strategies for reducing the overuse of antibiotics is vaccination. Vaccines can prevent infections from occurring first, thereby reducing the need for antibiotic treatments. This is particularly important in the fight against AMR. By preventing bacterial infections, vaccines limit the conditions that often lead to the misuse or overuse of antibiotics.

mRNA vaccine technology, which was developed during the COVID-19 pandemic, has potential not only for preventing viral diseases but also for tailoring vaccines to bacterial infections, further reducing antibiotic dependency.

1.6   Sustainability

Sustainability in infection prevention goes beyond reducing antibiotic use. Nurses, as frontline healthcare workers, are in a prime position to lead these efforts by advocating for the efficient use of personal protective equipment (PPE), supporting sustainable practices in waste management, and promoting preventive measures such as vaccination to reduce overall resource consumption. A commitment to sustainability will be essential in making healthcare systems more resilient to future pandemics.

Robust infection prevention and control (IPC) programs are central to building resilient, responsive, and sustainable health systems. These programs align with the United Nations' Sustainable Development Goals (SDGs), reduce health costs, and provide safer healthcare for all. However, paradoxically, IPC programs themselves contribute to health sector emissions, waste generation, and ecosystem contamination [7].

A key aspect of sustainability is reducing the broader ecological footprint of healthcare practices. For example, PPE is vital for preventing the spread of infections, but the pandemic revealed the environmental and logistical challenges associated with PPE shortages, overuse, and waste management. In addition to PPE, wastewater treatment and the safe disposal of pharmaceutical waste are important considerations in ensuring long-term sustainability.

Nurses must lead efforts to develop and implement sustainable infection control practices. This includes advocating for the efficient use of PPE, promoting vaccinations to prevent infections, and supporting healthcare innovations that minimize environmental impact. Nurses face the dual challenge of maintaining effective infection control while advancing environmental sustainability. Achieving this balance is essential to ensuring that healthcare systems remain resilient and capable of responding to future pandemics and public health crises.

1.7 Healthcare Staff

In the face of growing infection control challenges, healthcare systems are facing a shortage of skilled professionals worldwide. The increasing demand for services, coupled with burnout and rising retirement rates among nurses, has brought critical momentum. To address the growing shortage of skilled healthcare professionals, particularly nurses, healthcare systems must prioritize not only recruitment but also retention strategies. Making nursing and infection prevention roles more appealing is one approach. This includes developing specialized training programs in areas such as antimicrobial resistance (AMR) and infection control, attracting new talent while equipping current nurses with the skills to confront these global challenges [8].

As infection control becomes more complex, nursing education must evolve to prepare the next generation for the challenges ahead. The development of a curriculum that includes simulation-based training, problem-based learning, and interdisciplinary case studies is vital for ensuring that nurses can collaborate effectively. Such training should emphasize communication skills, shared decision-making, and the ability to adapt to complex, rapidly evolving clinical situations [9, 10].

Programs aimed at combating AMR should adopt teaching strategies and methods that foster the development of interprofessional skills among nurses. Collaborative practice ensures that nurses can work effectively within interdisciplinary teams to make critical decisions, from implementing antimicrobial stewardship programs to responding to infection outbreaks.

Continuing education will also be crucial to keep nurses updated on advancements in infection prevention and control, including AI-driven monitoring systems, new antimicrobials, and vaccines. Nurses need to embrace lifelong learning and continually update their knowledge and skills to meet the dynamic demands of infection control.

Relational leadership practices should be supported to enhance job satisfaction, retention, and productivity within healthcare settings, creating a positive work environment that promotes nurse well-being and professional growth [11].

Infection prevention is not just the responsibility of healthcare workers—it requires a whole-of-society approach. Public education and health literacy are essential to empowering individuals to take charge of their own health. According to the One Health approach, the health of humans, animals, and the environment is interconnected.

AMR is a global threat that does not respect borders, and it will require international cooperation. The UN General Assembly High-Level Meeting on AMR reaffirmed that governments, healthcare systems, and industries must work together to develop new antibiotics, vaccines, and diagnostic tools while also ensuring equitable access to these life-saving resources across all income levels [4].

1.8   Conclusion

The future of infection prevention and control involves innovation, education, and collaboration. Artificial Intelligence (AI) and advanced analytics will continue to transform how infections are monitored. But these tools require the leadership and wise decision-making of skilled healthcare professionals, particularly nurses, to effectively guide the response. They will remain the bedrock of infection control and translate data into action.

Challenges in infection prevention and control—from AMR to the need for sustainable healthcare practices—will require innovative and adaptable approaches. The next generation of nurses will need to include not only skilled caregivers but also leaders in public health, educators, critical thinkers, and advocates for sustainable, collaborative, and evidence-based practices. For all these reasons, the next generation of nurses must be prepared to take on multifaceted roles. They will not only be skilled caregivers but also act as leaders in public health, educators, critical thinkers, and champions of sustainable healthcare practices. Through advanced training and the integration of new technologies, nurses will continue to address infection control challenges, particularly antimicrobial resistance, and ensure the resilience of global health systems.

References

1. Hassoun-Kheir N, Guedes M, Ngo Nsoga MT, Argante L, Arieti F, Gladstone BP, et al. A systematic review on the excess health risk of antibiotic-resistant bloodstream infections for six key pathogens in Europe. Clin Microbiol Infect. 2024;30:S14–25.
2. WHO Director-General's opening remarks at the multi-stakeholder panel, high level meeting on AMR—26 September 2024 [Internet]. [Cited 2024 Sep 27]. Available from https://www. who.int/director-general/speeches/detail/who-director-general-s-opening-remarks-at-the-multi-stakeholder-panel%2D%2Dhigh-level-meeting-on-amr%2D%2D-26-september-2024

3. Naghavi M, Vollset SE, Ikuta KS, Swetschinski LR, Gray AP, Wool EE, et al. Global burden of bacterial antimicrobial resistance 1990–2021: a systematic analysis with forecasts to 2050. Lancet. 2024;S0140673624018671

4. Letter from President General Assembly on AMR Political Declaration | General Assembly of the United Nations [Internet]. [Cited 2024 Sep 29]. Available from https://www.un.org/pga/78/2024/05/21/letter-from-president-general-assembly-on-amr-political-declaration/

5. Zay Ya K, Win PTN, Bielicki J, Lambiris M, Fink G. Association between antimicrobial stewardship programs and antibiotic use globally: a systematic review and meta-analysis. JAMA Netw Open. 2023;6(2):e2253806.

6. Delivery of antimicrobial stewardship competencies in UK pre-registration nurse education programmes: a national cross-sectional survey—ScienceDirect [Internet]. [Cited 2024 Sep 28]. Available from https://www.sciencedirect.com/science/article/abs/pii/S0195670121004229

7. Saravanos GL, Islam MS, Huang Y, Basseal JM, Seale H, Mitchell BG, et al. Infection prevention and control programme priorities for sustainable health and environmental systems. BMC Glob Public Health. 2024;2(1):6.

8. Yasin YM, Alomari A, Al-Hamad A, Kehyayan V. The impact of COVID-19 on nurses' job satisfaction: a systematic review and meta-analysis. Front Public Health. 2024;11:1285101.

9. Corvetto MA, Altermatt FR, Belmar F, Escudero E. Health care simulation as a training tool for epidemic management: a systematic review. Simul Healthc. 2023;18(6):382.

10. Brazil V, Reedy G. Translational simulation revisited: an evolving conceptual model for the contribution of simulation to healthcare quality and safety. Adv Simul. 2024;9(1):16.

11. Cummings GG, Tate K, Lee S, Wong CA, Paananen T, Micaroni SPM, et al. Leadership styles and outcome patterns for the nursing workforce and work environment: a systematic review. Int J Nurs Stud. 2018;85:19–60.

Introduction to Infection Prevention and Control: From Florence Nightingale to the Present

2

Elisa Fabbri

2.1   Introduction

"Nursing, more than any other profession, is a progressive calling. Year after year, nurses must learn new and better methods as medicine, surgery, and hygiene improve. Year after year, nurses are called to do more and better than they have in the past." [1]. With these words, in the 1800s, Florence Nightingale began and founded modern nursing, revolutionizing the view of the nurse in society by approaching care with a scientific method and employing adequately trained and paid nurses for healthcare services.

To speak about modern Nursing as a profession, it is necessary to step back in time and trace the key milestones that have shaped the history of nurses. The shift from the figure of the mother-caregiver to Florence Nightingale's insights was not brief, and the profession still today seeks social, cultural, economic, and occupational recognition, which is slow to materialize. The concept of *ad-sistere* (to stand beside) is historically tied to the figure of the woman, mother-companion-caregiver. In the history of care, two distinct paths emerged early on: the "cure," reserved for the male figure of the doctor, and the "care," reserved for women, especially mothers.

With the advent of Christianity, the focus on others increased, and deaconesses were the first to promote care as a religious vocation. Patients began to be categorized based on their conditions and care needs, and nurses, both religious and secular, were required to know not only the sacred scriptures but also the basics of various diseases and the medications used to treat them. It was the Humanism-inspired revolution that brought the concepts of health and disease closer together through a scientific approach. Starting from the 1600s, with the flourishing of new medical and scientific discoveries, new theories and conceptions about health

E. Fabbri (✉)
IPC Nurse, Emilia-Romagna, Italy

© The Author(s), under exclusive license to Springer Nature Switzerland AG 2025
B. Oomen, S. Gastaldi (eds.), *Principles of Nursing Infection Prevention Control*,
Principles of Specialty Nursing, https://doi.org/10.1007/978-3-031-84469-0_2

emerged: clinical doctors introduced the first classifications of diseases based on the observation of signs and symptoms conducted at the patient's bedside. Disease became a phenomenon that needed to be studied like any other natural phenomenon, and from this era, doctors relied on their perceptual skills, intuition, and accumulated experience, aided by the first diagnostic instruments.

In the eighteenth century, scientific progress led to the dominance of doctors, under whose strict control nurses were relegated to purely hotel services and night watch duties. The real turning point for the nursing profession is linked to the intervention of Florence Nightingale (1820–1910), an English noblewoman with a strong religious vocation, who was the first to be properly credited with the title of "nurse."

During the Crimean War of 1853, Nightingale, along with 39 other nurses she had selected, took charge of the English military hospital at Scutari, despite initial distrust from the doctors. By applying a new organizational method that ensured, first and foremost, the hygiene of the therapeutic environment, she managed to significantly reduce mortality rates and was one of the first to understand the importance of epidemiology and medical statistics in interpreting information on disease progression and the effectiveness of care provided.

Returning home as a heroine, she founded the Nightingale School and Home for Nurses in London in 1860, using public funds raised for her work in Crimea. Her main contribution to the professionalization of nursing was in the area of education: with the goal of raising the social status of nurses, she recognized the importance of their ability to lead and teach others. She selected the first 15 nurses from the school attached to St. Thomas Hospital, women of noble standing and impeccable behavior, and sent them abroad to spread the "Nightingale model." She mandated that the students reside in a dormitory where they were molded in both technique and character by the strict discipline of the director.

In the organization envisioned by the Nightingale Schools, there was no interference between the work of doctors and that of nurses, as their respective roles were clearly defined. The Nightingale training system aimed for the nurse to achieve mastery in technical competence and moral conduct. In 1859, she also wrote "Notes on Nursing," the first modern textbook for nursing care. She collaborated with Elizabeth Blackwell, the first woman to earn a medical degree in the United States, to establish the Woman's Medical College in their homeland, England. She received many honors, and in 2020 (postponed to 2021 and 2022 due to the COVID-19 pandemic), the 200th anniversary of her birth was celebrated worldwide [2].

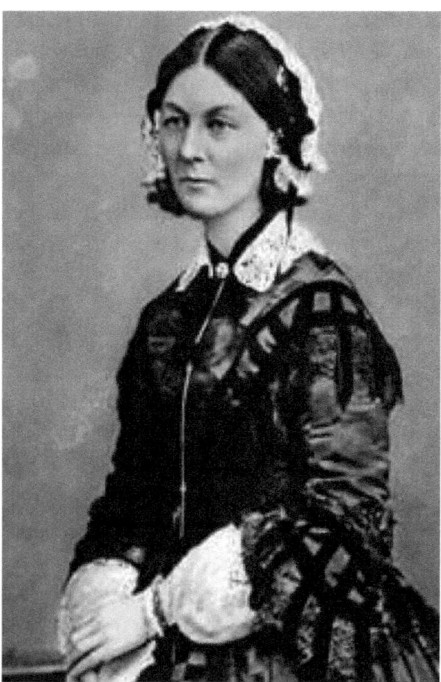

With her, the concept of disease and health was introduced for the first time, and it became clear that nurses needed to attend a course to earn the title and possess both foundational and advanced knowledge to ensure safe environments and provide adequate care. Florence Nightingale was the first nursing theorist, initiating a dynamic process of redefining the role of nurses, based on the evolution of clinical practice, technology, and ongoing research, a process that continues to this day.

2.2   Evolution of Nursing in Infection Prevention and Control (IPC)

2.2.1   Definition of Infection Prevention

Infection prevention and control (IPC) is a discipline in which epidemiologic and statistical principles are used in order to prevent or control the incidence and prevalence of infection. The primary role of an IPC program is to reduce the risk of acquisition of hospital-acquired infection, thereby protecting both patients and staff from adverse infection-related outcomes. In order to ensure that an infection control program is successful, the appropriate infrastructure and institutional support, both material and administrative, needs to be made available to hospital epidemiology staff [3].

There are two main IPC areas of concern within health and social care, and these are healthcare associated infections (HAIs) and antimicrobial resistance (AMR).

Infection control is an essential process of any health care organization. It deals with factors related to the spread of infections among patients, among staff, and between patients and staff. It includes preventive measures such as hand washing, cleaning, disinfection, sterilization, and vaccination. Other aspects include monitoring and managing outbreaks of infection and investigating their causes, and last but not least, prescribing antibiotics correctly in the right time, manner, and molecule.

2.2.1.1 Evolution of Nursing in IPC

Nursing and midwifery activities are essential elements of all national health systems. Nurses and midwives have been providing care for a long time and constitute the majority of healthcare personnel in many countries worldwide. Their importance has been recognized by the World Health Organization (WHO) since its founding in 1948.

The evolution of the nurse specializing in infection prevention has developed at different times and in different ways across nations, depending on the organizational, regulatory, and educational context of each country.

The International Council of Nurses (ICN), founded in 1899, was the first and largest international organization for health professionals, laying the foundation for a series of developments that have fueled WHO policies and activities related to nursing care. The founding of the WHO not only highlighted the role of nurses but also brought the attention of politicians and diplomats to the importance of nursing care.

In the United States, the hospital discipline of infection control was established in the 1950s in response to a national outbreak of nosocomial *Staphylococcus aureus* infections and the recognition of the need for surveillance of nosocomial infections [4]. However, the concept of epidemiology and infection prevention has its roots in an earlier period, when in 1846, Hungarian physician Semmelweis noted that mortality from puerperal fever among women who gave birth with midwives was lower than that of mothers whose children were delivered by doctors. After conducting a thorough analysis of the differences between the groups, Semmelweis concluded that the high rate of puerperal fever was caused by cadaveric material on the hands of medical students who came to the obstetric clinic directly from the autopsy room. A policy of handwashing with chlorinated lime solution was introduced before contact with the mother, and the mortality rate among mothers attended by doctors drastically decreased [5].

The initial priorities of WHO's action was the treatment of widespread infectious diseases in many countries, such as malaria, tuberculosis, venereal diseases, maternal and child health, and environmental hygiene. These were quickly followed by issues related to the healthcare system, such as the administration of public health and ensuring medical and nursing care. For nursing, the delegations of Ireland and the United States were the first to request the establishment of posts and the allocation of funds to organize an expert committee, making it clear to the international community the importance of nursing care in making a difference in people's lives.

In the 1970s, the concept of proactive medicine emerged, promoting preventive activities by multidisciplinary teams with specific expertise, eventually leading to the formation of specialized teams for different diseases. In the 1980s, specific nursing competencies were developed through the dissemination of well-defined study programs with both basic and advanced knowledge. This opened up the possibility of organizing nursing functions at various levels in different national health systems, in international organizations, and initiated nursing research. From this point on, nurses began to specialize in specific clinical areas and based on the development of specific health evolutions, such as the global alarm in the mid-1990s regarding antimicrobial resistance and infectious diseases. This led to the emergence of nurses specializing in the prevention of healthcare-associated infections (HAIs) and in the fight against antimicrobial resistance (AMR) [6].

The dissemination of nurses specializing in HAI prevention and AMR control varies across nations and is influenced by political choices and national regulations. However, the activities and skills required of specialist nurses are shared:

- Participating in the definition of health policies at local, national, and international levels.
- Planning, managing, and evaluating IPC and AMR interventions in collaboration with other professionals involved, both in hospitals and community settings.
- Collaborating on and promoting research, training, and innovative projects within the specific field.
- Providing evidence-based support and consultations to all clinicians in need.
- Using effective communication techniques and facilitating the exchange of information and training with healthcare professionals, patients, and caregivers.
- Adapting and facilitating the use of new technologies in clinical care processes.
- Promoting cultural change in IPC and AMR prevention, control, and contrast.
- Keeping their own knowledge and skills up to date.

In May 2022, the seventy-fifth World Health Assembly adopted a global strategy for the prevention and control of infections (IPC) [7], which called for the implementation of accredited IPC curricula at all levels of healthcare training.

In response to this, the WHO drafted a curriculum [8] that provides a comprehensive framework to improve IPC practices among those responsible for developing learning resources and overseeing training within healthcare organizations. The holistic approach involves a wide range of personnel, from clinical staff to administrative and auxiliary services, ensuring an inclusive approach to IPC training. It outlines three distinct levels of competence within the curriculum:

- *Basic*: Introduces universal basic IPC principles applicable to all healthcare roles.
- *Intermediate*: Provides more detailed IPC practices, particularly for clinical professionals in direct patient contact.
- *Advanced*: Offers specialized IPC knowledge tailored to clinical specialists and management roles, reflecting the specific needs of their positions and contexts.

This reference tool is essential for supporting the planning, development, and localization of IPC educational materials, aligning closely with the WHO's core components for IPC programs and the recommendations outlined in the global strategy and action plan on IPC. It supports countries in their efforts to implement actions aimed at improving IPC knowledge and skills among healthcare and care staff, in line with the recommendations of the WHO global action plan and monitoring framework. It enhances the IPC competencies of healthcare and care professionals and strengthens the healthcare system's ability to manage and prevent infections effectively, promoting safer healthcare environments, even in the context of epidemics, pandemics, and other public health emergencies.

2.3 Conclusion

The evolution of nursing and the progressive specialization have allowed nurses to adapt their practices to the developments in clinical, technological, and organizational aspects of healthcare. This has led to the implementation and improvement of activities within hospitals and the initiation and structuring of activities in community settings.

Specialized nurses in IPC and AMR play a multifunctional role in improving patient safety and public health. Their expertise is crucial for preventing infections and helping to combat AMR, especially as healthcare systems face new challenges posed by emerging pathogens and global health crises.

Having a national policy and a curriculum to support the training of healthcare workers in infection prevention and control and providing this training to all frontline healthcare workers and cleaners (upon hiring in all facilities at minimum, and annually in tertiary care hospitals), are minimum requirements for all countries to ensure safe care and adequate preparedness for epidemics [9]. Training and education, including hand hygiene, are among the eight core components identified by the WHO to achieve effective infection prevention and control programs at both the national and facility levels [10].

However, the progress of countries in implementing training programs and assessing their effects remains insufficient. WHO's global surveys on infection prevention and control programs conducted between 2017 and 2022 consistently showed that training and education scored the lowest, indicating gaps in the preparedness for effective infection prevention and control implementation [11, 12].

In 2023, all countries committed to adopting the new global strategy for infection prevention and control, which includes a fundamental strategic direction on training and education.

This strategy not only calls for integrating infection prevention and control into the entire healthcare education system through the development of pre-service, postgraduate, and in-service training programs but also supports the creation of local competencies in infection prevention and control and recognized career paths for infection prevention and control professionals, alongside the development of educational resources for patients and families.

Building on these commitments, and given the growing threats posed by healthcare-associated infections, antimicrobial resistance, and emerging infections, World Hand Hygiene Day 2024 provided a unique platform for all healthcare workers, infection prevention and control professionals, policymakers, decision-makers, and the public to engage and act. It offered a range of resources to support these efforts. The proposed approach supports a shift towards continuous, practical, and experiential learning that engages healthcare workers, moving beyond the mere acquisition of theoretical knowledge. Innovative training methods, including those that value the unique experiences of healthcare workers and the use of games and other technologies (such as WHO's new hand hygiene game) [13], are strongly encouraged. Integrating infection prevention and control training within clinical practice, continuous education, and periodic assessment to ensure knowledge retention and effectiveness are fundamental for progress. By seizing this opportunity, all those who influence better and safer healthcare environments can forge a path toward a more resilient healthcare workforce and a more equitable and sustainable future for global healthcare, better prepared for epidemics and safeguarding the well-being of both healthcare workers and patients.

This text aims to delve deeper into the topics that have been briefly listed and described in this introduction, attempting to contextualize them within various care settings and illustrating their application in daily practice.

We hope that all readers will find in the following paragraphs useful insights and further explorations that can be extended to their own work contexts, contributing to the ongoing spread of a stronger culture of IPC prevention and the fight against AMR.

References

1. Lippi D, Borghi L. La penna di Florence Nightingale. Firenze: Pontecorboli editore; 2020.
2. Rocco G, Cipolla C, Stievano A. La storia del nursing in Italia e nel contesto internazionale. FrancoAngeli. p. 97. ISBN 9788891723147
3. Royal College of Nursing. The role of the link nurse in infection prevention and control (IPC): developing a link nurse framework. Review in February 2023; 2021.
4. Scheckler WE, Brimhall D, Buck AS. Requirements for infrastructure and essential activities of infection control and epidemiology in hospitals: a consensus panel report. Society for Healthcare Epidemiology of America. Infect Control Hosp Epidemiol. 1998;19(2):114–24. [PubMed] [Google Scholar] [Ref list]
5. Noakes TD, Borresen J, Hew-Butler T, Lambert MI, Jordaan E. Semmelweis and the aetiology of puerperal sepsis 160 years on: an historical review. Epidemiol Infect. 2008;136(1):1–9. [PMC free article] [PubMed] [Google Scholar] [Ref list]
6. World Health Organization. Nursing and midwifery in the history of the World Health Organization (1948–2017). ISBN 978-92-4-151190-2; 2017.
7. World Health Organization. Global strategy on infection prevention and control. ISBN 978-92-4-008051-5; 2023.
8. World Health Organization. Infection prevention and control in-service education and training curriculum. ISBN 978-92-4-009412-3; 2024.
9. WHO. Minimum requirements for infection prevention and control programmes. https://www.who.int/publications/i/item/9789241516945. Accessed 26 Sept 2024.

10. WHO. Guidelines on core components of infection prevention and control programmes at the national and acute health care facility level. Geneva: World Health Organization; 2016.
11. Tomczyk S, Twyman A, de Kraker MEA, et al. The first WHO global survey on infection prevention and control in health-care facilities. Lancet Infect Dis. 2022;22:845–56.
12. WHO. Global report on infection prevention and control. Geneva: World Health Organization; 2022.
13. WHO. My 5 moments for hand hygiene. https://5mgame.lxp.academy.who.int/. Accessed 26 Sept 2024.

The Vital Role of Nurses in IPC

3

Tihana Gašpert

3.1 Empowering Nurses as Frontline Defenders: The Critical Role of Infection Prevention, Specialized Training, and Patient Safety

For an infection to be transmitted, there must be a source of infection, a method of transmission, and a host that is susceptible to the infection. Implementing basic precautions for all patients is a crucial measure in preventing the transfer of infectious organisms, as nurses cannot determine which patients may be infected or colonized [1–4]. Standard precautions are implemented to safeguard nurses and patients by preventing the transmission of pathogens, whether it is through direct contact between individuals, contact with contaminated surfaces, or exposure to contaminated environments [5].

Transporting patients within a facility can potentially provide chances for the spread of infection. Nurses have the potential to contaminate elevator controls or door handles. If these surfaces are not cleaned, they can serve as an indirect source of infectious organisms for other patients, visitors, or healthcare workers. This can lead to infection or the transmission of infection to another person or surface [4]. Nurses employ droplet precautions while caring for patients confirmed or suspected to be ill with diseases that are spread through respiratory droplets produced by coughing, sneezing, or speaking. Droplet precautions involve the utilization of personal protective equipment (PPE), such as a surgical mask, and the application of a mask on the patient while being transported [6].

Healthcare staff employ airborne precautions when providing care for patients who are confirmed or suspected to be infected with infections that are transferred through the air. Airborne precautions involve the use of PPE. It also includes placing

T. Gašpert (✉)
University Hospital Rijeka, Rijeka, Croatia

Faculty of Health Sciences, University of Maribor, Maribor, Slovenia

a mask on the patient during transportation and using environmental controls [4]. Nurses implement and enforce preventive measures to reduce the risk of infection by leading in hand hygiene and PPE compliance. As role models, they set the standard for proper hand hygiene and PPE use, encouraging others to follow suit [6].

3.1.1 Patient Safety

Patient safety, as defined by the World Health Organization, refers to the absence of avoidable injury to patients and the prevention of unnecessary harm by healthcare workers [7]. The concept of a safety culture is dynamic and centers upon the prevention of medical errors and the preservation of patient safety [8], which include efficient communication, adequate staffing, adherence to procedures, environmental safety and security, a culture that promotes safety, supportive leadership, comprehensive orientation and training, and transparent communication regarding medical errors [7, 9]. The primary goal of this system is to consistently and continuously minimize risks, decrease the frequency of preventable harm, reduce the likelihood of errors, and mitigate the consequences of harm when it does occur [7].

The primary responsibility of nurses is to ensure patient safety and minimize the risk of harm while delivering care in various healthcare settings, including both short-term and long-term care facilities [10, 11]. Nurses strive to deliver comprehensive nursing care to patients, encompassing the promotion of health and well-being, prevention of infections, and therapeutic nursing care within healthcare organizations and the community [12]. Nurses are required to follow the organizational methods for recognizing potential dangers and hazards by evaluating the patient, devising a care plan, conducting monitoring and surveillance activities, verifying information, providing assistance, and communicating with other healthcare professionals [13–15]. For interventions aimed at preventing practice errors and achieving sustainable and safer healthcare systems, nurses must adhere to patient safety principles, along with clear policies, leadership, research-driven safety initiatives, training of healthcare staff, and patient participation [7, 15–17].

Standard precautions refer to the necessary measures that must be implemented to prevent the transmission of infection between individuals or from contaminated surfaces when there is a likelihood of encountering blood, bodily fluids, secretions, and excretions like urine and feces [18, 19]. Standard precautions are essential measures employed to prevent the transmission of infectious agents during interactions between nurses and patients in any healthcare setting. These precautions aim to prevent infections from spreading from nurses to patients and vice versa [20–22]. These practices include hand hygiene, proper use of personal protective equipment, safe administration of patient injections, proper handling of contaminated equipment and patient environments, as well as respiratory hygiene [22].

Nurses bear the duty of safeguarding their health to prevent jeopardizing patient safety. They can significantly impact the likelihood of patients developing infections [23, 24]. Strict adherence to established procedures is mandatory in the healthcare sector as it forms the foundation for infection control strategies and ensures safety [25]. Following these principles is essential to maintain an infection-free environment and minimize the risk of infection [7, 24].

The Universal Protection Framework by Sands et al. [26] is a comprehensive strategy that includes four interconnected areas, reinforced by communication and education:

1. Fundamental infection prevention measures: implementing universal masking for all individuals (staff, visitors, and patients), utilizing personal protective equipment, ensuring environmental safety, and establishing specific policies and procedures for providing care to patients based on infectious disease.
2. Control of access: information regarding visitation, personnel screening, and physical security.
3. Distancing: providing guidelines about the implementation of social distancing measures, the arrangement of public areas, and the grouping of patients.
4. Flow of patients. The primary concern is the supervision of patients as they move through the facility to reduce the likelihood of exposure to risks.

An often-employed approach is the reduction of superfluous workflow. The restriction on visitors, for example, results in increased efficiency in providing care by eliminating the usual disruptions caused by excessive traffic. The decrease in access also facilitates enhanced control and surveillance of personnel entering the premises, thus lowering the risk of exposure. The implementation of fundamental infection prevention measures focuses on ensuring good hand hygiene and surface cleaning [26].

3.1.2   Infection Prevention and Control for Nurses

Infection prevention and control refers to the implementation of systematic procedures, policies, and protocols aimed at minimizing the likelihood of infections [27]. These strategies aim to create a safe environment by implementing protocols that decrease the probability of transmission of infectious agents. Infection in healthcare institutions is a major cause of illness and death, and it is a problem that affects the entire world [28].

Healthcare-associated infections (HAIs), also referred to as hospital-acquired infections, are infections that patients acquire while undergoing medical treatment at a healthcare facility, such as a hospital or clinic. These infections can be caused by bacteria, viruses, fungi, or parasites and can present in a variety of ways, ranging from benign to severe [29]. Within the healthcare ecosystem, nurses are the primary and most frequent line of defense against infections. They are at the forefront of efforts to prevent infections due to their unique role, which is defined by continuous and direct patient care. The multifaceted nature of their responsibilities helps to ensure the deliverance of secure and effective care, which also reduces the potential transmission of infectious agents [30].

The prevention of infections is contingent upon the maintenance of proper hand hygiene. Consistent and appropriate hand hygiene has been shown to have a substantial impact on the containment of pathogens in healthcare settings, despite its straightforward concept. Numerous studies have demonstrated that the transmission of infectious agents and, consequently, the incidence of infections can be significantly reduced by adhering to recommended hand hygiene practices [31].

However, nurses are responsible for a much more extensive role in infection prevention than merely administering direct care. Nurse educators are essential in educating patients and their families about the importance of implementing infection prevention measures. By offering advice on the maintenance of indwelling medical devices, instructing patients on wound care after discharge, and emphasizing the significance of hand hygiene, nurses empower patients to become informed participants in their recovery and care [32].

Furthermore, nurses frequently participate in collaborative endeavors with infection perfectionists and other members of the healthcare team. They remain informed about the most recent evidence-based practices in the field of infection control by participating in regular training sessions, discussions, and meetings [33].

The criticality of nurses' responsibilities in infection prevention has been further underscored by the increasing prevalence of antibiotic-resistant bacteria. To mitigate the issue of antibiotic resistance, nurses implement a variety of approaches, such as administering antibiotics precisely, educating patients on the importance of finishing antibiotic courses, and guaranteeing that patients receive the appropriate dosage at the prescribed intervals [34, 35].

Nurses are the foundation of infection prevention due to their dedication, expertise, and meticulous attention to detail. They ensure that healthcare facilities remain secure retreats for recuperation and restoration in their capacity as advocates for patient health. The healthcare environment is constantly evolving, and dynamic, as new pathogens are discovered and established ones develop resistance. It is imperative that healthcare professionals, particularly nurses who are in direct contact with patients, remain informed about the most effective infection prevention methods. This requirement underscores the importance of ongoing education and training, which ensures that all nurses have the requisite knowledge and skills to protect both themselves and their patients [16, 34, 35].

Nurses have a significant responsibility for preventing the spread of infections. In addition, they have a significant responsibility in patient education and ensuring that all aspects of their nursing practice are based on the latest scientific research. Nurses possess a unique potential to facilitate change and enhance the standards of patient care when they serve as advisors to patients. Nurses can utilize much equipment to provide patients with a secure environment. Hand hygiene is the paramount nursing intervention for preventing infections, and it is a powerful tool in the nurse's arsenal [36].

Nurses may demonstrate leadership in managing and preventing the transmission of infections in any situation and adhere to strict patient safety protocols by utilizing their expertise, skills, and discernment to execute efficient and prompt infection control procedures. It is imperative to prioritize infection control in hospitals to protect patients, healthcare personnel, and visitors:

- Hand hygiene. Ensuring proper hand hygiene is essential for preventing and minimizing the spread of diseases. An effective method to prevent the spread of infection is thorough handwashing. Posters highlighting the importance of proper hand hygiene should be displayed adjacent to sinks and antiseptic materials. According to the WHO "Five Moments" model, nurses are advised to wash their hands before and after interacting with a patient, before carrying out a clean or aseptic procedure, following any potential exposure to bodily fluids, and after touching the patient's immediate environment or belongings.
- Personal protective equipment (PPE). Nurses must utilize suitable PPE, including gloves, gowns, masks, and eye protection while delivering patient care to avoid the transmission of infectious organisms. PPE is used to create a physical barrier between nurses and potentially infectious items.
- Ensuring cleanliness is crucial for healthcare facilities as it contributes to a pleasant and secure environment, ultimately leading to higher patient satisfaction. Regular cleaning and disinfection of hospital rooms, equipment, and surfaces is necessary to avoid the transmission of infections. Proper disinfectants and cleaning products help prevent cross-contamination.
- Isolation and screening. Screening and isolating individuals colonized or infected with multidrug-resistant organisms (MDRO) is necessary to prevent the transmission of the sickness to other patients. To prevent the spread of contagious illnesses, individuals who are known or suspected to be infected are segregated from others through the implementation of isolation protocols.
- Education. Ensuring nurses receive ongoing education and training on infection control measures is crucial to keep them up to date with the most effective methods. Understanding the transmission pathway, the modes of illness dissemination, and efficient preventive strategies are all integral components of this. Training should include the coverage of standard precautions, which are the essential infection control procedures administered to all patients.
- Sanitization and Decontamination. Before usage, it is imperative to clean or sterilize all medical equipment, especially those that can be reused, to prevent the transmission of diseases. Sterilization is typically employed when essential medical equipment meets sterile body parts. Disinfection refers to the process of decreasing the quantity of microorganisms on surfaces, tools, or in the surrounding environment to a level that is considered safe.
- Surveillance and Documentation. Hospitals must promptly detect and report instances of contagious disease outbreaks and promptly implement the requisite steps to control their spread. An effective monitoring system is characterized by its ability to compare, anticipate, and concentrate on achieving predetermined targets. Reporting involves transmitting surveillance data to the appropriate authorities or groups responsible for monitoring and implementing infection control protocols.

- Vaccination. Nurses must receive immunization against infectious diseases to effectively prevent the transmission of sickness. Nurses are required to undergo vaccines to protect their well-being and prevent the acquisition and transmission of diseases. To provide effective infection control in the hospital environment, nurses must comply with local rules and stay updated on immunization guidelines provided by their employers and public health authorities.
- Adherence and Conformity. To ensure compliance and effective monitoring, organizations should implement the following essential measures. Organizations should establish explicit policies and procedures that delineate the exact measures nurses must undertake to prevent and manage infections. These regulations must undergo periodic evaluation and modification, and they should be founded upon the latest recommendations substantiated by research. All nurses must undergo infection prevention training. This directive necessitates multiple training sessions, continuous education, reminders, and feedback on compliance. This may involve performing audits, evaluating surveillance data, and obtaining input from employees. Establishing and maintaining effective communication channels with patients, guests, and medical personnel can help identify problem areas and encourage compliance with infection control protocols.

3.1.3 Training for Nurses

The education and training of healthcare personnel are crucial in implementing methods and processes to decrease infection rates [12]. Attending education allows nurses to acquire the necessary theoretical and practical knowledge to develop specific abilities and engage in ongoing professional development [22]. In addition, the use of evidence-based information is essential for ensuring patient safety and delivering high-quality care, ultimately leading to improved patient outcomes [25]. Nurses, as integral members of the healthcare team, have a significant impact on the transmission of infections and are crucial in the management and control of infection prevention. Hence, nurses must possess accurate, current, and relevant scientific knowledge about different types of hospital infections, their impact on affected patients, the mortality rate, the escalation in expenses, and the identification of individuals at risk, as well as the guidelines for prevention [37]. A higher level of nurses' knowledge has a positive impact on their performance [38, 39].

Numerous institutions are presently incorporating simulation-based training in conjunction with traditional classroom-based learning. The implementation of simulation exercises can considerably improve the practical skills required for infection prevention and the retention of information [40, 41].

The emergence of online learning modules and platforms has opened an additional avenue for education. Nurses can participate in self-paced learning and examine the material at their leisure, as digital platforms provide a high degree of adaptability. The adoption of e-learning modules related to infection prevention has experienced a significant increase. These modules improve the comprehension and adherence of healthcare professionals to infection control protocols. The importance of interdisciplinary training sessions is expanding beyond the realm of individual education. These interactions can help to address knowledge gaps and ensure that all members of the healthcare team share the same perspective on infection prevention. Furthermore, audit and continuous feedback systems are essential in the field of education. Academic institutions can evaluate the effectiveness of their instructional initiatives, identify areas that require improvement, and make necessary modifications by implementing consistent evaluations and feedback mechanisms. The quality and effectiveness of infection prevention education can be significantly enhanced through the implementation of iterative feedback mechanisms [42].

3.1.4   The Effectiveness of Teamwork and Dialogue in the Prevention of Infections

It is impossible to attribute effective infection prevention to a single entity; it is a collaborative endeavor that requires the involvement of professionals and departments from a variety of disciplines. To guarantee that all nurses have the necessary knowledge to protect patients, information must be effortlessly transferred. Healthcare facilities that prioritized robust interdisciplinary collaboration experienced significantly lower rates of healthcare-associated infections than those that maintained departmental segregation. To deliberate, plan, and execute infection control measures, the convergence of expertise from various disciplines leads to more comprehensive and effective resolutions [43].

Additionally, communication and collaboration are not limited by the confines of institutions. Due to the global nature of health hazards, hospitals, research institutions, public health agencies, and even nations are obligated to exchange information, strategies, and insights. However, it is imperative to establish a culture that prioritizes communication and collaboration to ensure the success of these endeavors [44].

Nurses educate patients about infection risks and preventive measures, ensuring understanding across diverse patient populations. They play a crucial role in surveillance and early diagnosis, acting as the first line of defense in recognizing early signs of infection and initiating timely response measures. Nurses also advocate for infection prevention on behalf of patients, ensuring their safety and well-being. Through collaboration with multidisciplinary teams, nurses foster a cooperative approach to infection prevention, working closely with other healthcare professionals to protect patient health [36].

3.1.5   Personal Protective Equipment

When nurses are likely to come into touch with blood, bodily fluids, or other potentially infectious substances, regulatory bodies mandate that they wear personal protective equipment (PPE) [5, 7, 24]. One aspect of transmission-based precautions is the proper donning and doffing of personal protective equipment. Infection can occur if personnel doff PPE improperly. It is important to wash one's hands before donning gloves and again after removing them. Hand hygiene is still necessary even when wearing gloves [4]. Nurses must use eye protection if there is a reasonable expectation of blood, other potentially infectious materials, or other splashes, sprays, splatter, or droplets [4, 5, 7, 24]. When gown, gloves, or eye protection are being used, the mask should be removed last [5].

Face shields, masks, mittens, and garments can prevent the transmission of infectious agents when used correctly. It is imperative to ensure that PPE is worn, replaced, and disposed of appropriately. Nurses are required to comply with rigorous protocols when donning and doffing PPE to mitigate the risk of contamination [5]. Aseptic procedures are essential for the prevention of infections, particularly when inserting catheters or treating incisions. It is impossible to overstate the importance of maintaining a sterilized environment, as numerous HAIs are caused by invasive procedures. To substantially reduce the risk of infection, nurses adhere to aseptic protocols to ensure the cleanliness of the surrounding environment, equipment, and instruments [45].

3.1.6   Contact Precautions

Nurses must employ contact precautions alongside routine precautions while delivering treatment to patients who are confirmed or suspected to be infected or colonized with diseases that can be spread through direct or indirect touch [24]. Contact precautions encompass the utilization of PPE, the adoption of precautions during patient transportation, the consideration of patient placement to reduce contact with other patients, and the implementation of thorough environmental cleaning procedures [4].

Utilizing specialized monitoring equipment or disposable devices can effectively hinder the transmission of infectious agents from a contaminated blood pressure cuff or pulse oximeter sensor to healthcare workers or other patients. In the given situation, the staff chose disposable equipment that stayed with the patient during the entire process of care [46].

When transporting a patient who is infected, healthcare workers should implement measures to minimize the risk of pathogen transmission to other patients, personnel, and visitors, as well as to prevent contamination of the environment [4, 7, 46]. The executives of the health care organization should establish a protocol for the utilization of PPE during transportation.

3.2 Nurses' Role in Environmental Hygiene: Ensuring a Clean and Safe Healthcare Environment Through Oversight, Education, and Patient Communication

Twenty-five years ago, there was a shift in global perception of hand hygiene, recognizing the crucial role hands play as primary carriers of diseases between patients in hospital environments. Indeed, hands in healthcare are frequently polluted and seldom cleaned on movable surfaces. Contamination can be dynamically transferred between surfaces and hands [47]. In the transmission chain, contaminated hands can serve as the last link, while contaminated surfaces can act as earlier connections. It is optimal to adhere to the World Health Organization (WHO) concept of "Clean Care is Safer Care," [9, 21, 28].

Using the acronym "HANDS," the Joint Commission proposed five essential strategies for enhancing hand hygiene (HH):

- H = "habit."
- A = "Active feedback,"
- N = "No One Excused,"
- D = "Data-driven,"
- S = "Systems." [48].

The objective of the strategy is to cultivate positive hand hygiene practices among healthcare workers (HCWs) so that they automatically wash their hands and maintain hand hygiene before and after patient care, as well as upon entering or exiting a patient care area. Nurse leaders must consistently remind their staff of the significance of adherence to HH through active feedback. Real-time performance data should be used by health administrators and administrative staff to evaluate and provide feedback on the HH practice. Hospital authorities should acknowledge the critical role of HH in the preservation of patient safety and care, and all staff members must adhere to the HH guidelines. A data-driven HH policy necessitates the strict and routine monitoring and recording of compliance, with the data collected being analyzed to identify and prioritize areas for development and enhancement. Furthermore, it is imperative to continue researching to generate novel concepts that will address challenges associated with the implementation of the most effective HH practice [48]. Systems imply that HH responsiveness is a system-wide endeavor, with rules and regulations concerning HH being enforced throughout the health system.

Because enhanced environmental cleaning and decontamination procedures are consistently combined with other treatments during outbreaks, it becomes challenging to accurately assess their specific impact. The process of cleaning involves five primary factors, which include the removal of soil and the disinfection and cleaning at a microbiological level. The components to consider include the specific product or intervention being used, the technique and equipment employed for application, the type of surface being cleaned, the amount of contamination in the environment, and the individuals responsible for environmental hygiene during the cleaning process. If any of these aspects are absent, the cleaning will inherently be subpar. Therefore, the implementation of a multimodal strategy that considers these variables is necessary to change cleaning practices. Even the most effective cleaning material is rendered ineffective if not administered appropriately, and highly skilled workers are rendered useless if the product they are employing is not effective against the specific pathogen that needs to be eliminated or destroyed [49].

3.3   Future Trends in Hospital Infection Control

Hospitals are employing machine learning (ML) and artificial intelligence (AI) to actively identify and prevent the transmission of diseases. These techniques possess the capability to identify patterns and forecast potential outbreaks. AI technology is used to identify diseases on surfaces and monitor employees' compliance with hand hygiene protocols. If any issues are detected, the system promptly alerts staff members to take appropriate action. Telemedicine has become an essential tool in combating infections due to its ability to enable remote monitoring and consultations. To mitigate the danger of transmission inside hospital environments, healthcare personnel can get advantages from remote training and instruction on infection control techniques. Hospitals are currently exploring advanced sanitation methods, such as electrostatic sprayers, UV light, and hydrogen peroxide vapor, to efficiently cleanse surfaces and equipment. These improvements optimize cost-effectiveness by improving cleaning efficiency while significantly reducing the need for extensive manpower. Environmental monitoring systems give real-time data on elements that affect infection control, such as temperature, humidity, and air quality. Hospitals utilize this data to identify potential sources of sickness and implement proactive measures. Antibiotic stewardship programs are crucial in the prevention of antibiotic-resistant illnesses. Hospitals are implementing comprehensive antimicrobial management plans to enhance the utilization of antibiotics and mitigate the likelihood of antibiotic-resistant illnesses. Hospitals are integrating infection control into broader patient safety initiatives, acknowledging its crucial role in ensuring overall patient safety. Efficient management of these programs necessitates prioritizing early detection, prompt action against outbreaks, and the avoidance of infections. Hospitals are recognizing that infection control is a collective responsibility and are promoting increased collaboration to prevent the transmission of infections. To accomplish this, healthcare organizations must engage in the exchange of resources, expertise, and best practices. The future of infection prevention is likely to be enhanced by the establishment of organized networks and increased cooperation. Hospitals are engaging patients in their care and providing them with education, recognizing the significance of patient involvement in infection prevention. Providing patients with information on infection management strategies significantly contributes to reducing healthcare-associated infections. Possible future trends and opportunities may have an impact on hospital infection control.

The pace of technological advancement is occurring at an unparalleled and rapidly increasing rate, surpassing the capacity of any single person, group, occupation, or society to comprehensively comprehend or integrate. Within this context, it is crucial to possess the ability to acquire new knowledge, foster a sense of inquisitiveness to seek further understanding, develop effective learning strategies, and have a clear awareness of one's knowledge gaps. To effectively carry out their work, IPC nurses should leverage their inherent abilities, such as their interdisciplinary mindset, ability to comprehend the overall situation, and skill in establishing connections across the intricate network of healthcare facilities along the continuum of care. Important areas to focus on may encompass information systems and patient care technology, diagnostic testing, telemedicine, and emerging environmental technologies [50].

3.4   Nurses' Crucial Role in Infection Data Reporting: Advancing Quality Improvement, Professional Development, and Best Practices in Infection Prevention

The infection prevention (IP) nurses' tasks and roles have evolved due to the complicated topography of the continually expanding healthcare setting. Infection prevention also considers the broader perspective of ensuring patient safety throughout the entire care process. This ensures that patients, regardless of where they receive healthcare, achieve the most favorable results. While key principles of infection prevention and control (IPC) are applicable across various healthcare settings, nurses working in specialty settings such as acute care, long-term care, critical access, ambulatory, home health, dialysis, or ambulatory surgery may encounter distinct patient safety challenges and require specific practice methods [50].

The Association for Professionals in Infection Control and Epidemiology (APIC) Competency Model incorporates the basic competencies of the Certification Board of Infection Control and Epidemiology, Inc. (CBIC) and the APIC Professional and Practice Standards (PPS) [51]. The APIC Competency Model outlines distinct areas for the development of forward-thinking skills, allowing enhancing careers and addressing crucial IPC requirements. The future-oriented competency domains aim to predict and actively incorporate advancements in the field [50].

3.4.1   The APIC Competency Model

The APIC Competency Model outlines the essential knowledge, abilities, and attitudes required for effective work performance and professional advancement. The model consists of competency domains and subdomains that are focused on future-oriented skills. The core tenet of the model is patient safety, as it is at the heart of IPC practice, prioritizing the well-being of patients throughout the whole care process [50]. These domains are specifically selected for the development of future-oriented intellectual property (IP) competency:

1. The act or ability of leading or guiding a group of individuals towards a common goal.
2. Expert Management.
3. Enhancement of quality.
4. Operations for the Prevention and Control of Infections.
5. Informatics for Infection Prevention and Control.
6. Investigation [50].

3.4.1.1 Domain of Leadership Competencies

IPC nurses employ leadership abilities to build a distinct vision for IPC programs throughout all stages of healthcare delivery. The goal is to produce and enhance the commitment, capabilities, methodologies, and resources that are needed to turn visions and plans into reality. Acquiring and honing these talents throughout their professional journey will equip nurses with the necessary qualifications for potential leadership roles that may emerge down the line [50].

3.4.1.2 Domain of Communication

Effective communication is a crucial leadership ability for infection prevention due to the intricate problems. Communication encompasses the transmission of information or concepts to individuals and collectives, utilizing verbal and nonverbal means such as language, symbols, data, social media platforms, active listening, body language, and behavioral exemplification. IPC nurses utilize an evidence-based strategy to persuade and encourage the desired behaviors and performance. Nurses must proactively consider possible obstacles to successful communication, which might manifest as physical, psychological, attitudinal, or hierarchical challenges. Proficiency in active listening is crucial, as is the recognition of nonverbal signals. Individuals should develop the skill of convincing and exerting influence on others by employing a calm and consistent approach to reaching an agreement, supported by correct information, analysis, and applicable reasoning. IPC nurses must assess the optimal approach for transmitting the message. The primary outcome of successful communication is the mitigation of risk, promotion of interdisciplinary collaboration, education of key stakeholders in infection prevention and control, and enhancement of patient outcomes [50].

3.4.1.3 Domain of Critical Thinking

IPC nurses engage in critical thinking by thoroughly analyzing available information to assess a problem or scenario and then employing their expertise, experience, facts, and evidence to devise innovative solutions. Above all, critical thinking entails that the individual does not unquestioningly adopt a process, policy, or practice just based on the reason that it has been traditionally followed [50].

3.4.1.4 Domain of Collaboration

Infection prevention and control encompasses various aspects of healthcare and frequently involves sectors that are regulated by their specific guidelines and criteria. Accomplishing this task necessitates having a keen understanding of the current circumstances, the ability to perceive and manage emotions effectively, and a long-term plan for success. On other occasions, collaboration may involve fostering cooperation and maximizing the contributions of others. Additionally, it could imply the ability to effectively navigate and discuss requirements inside the broader framework of the group or institution. Effective collaboration necessitates various sorts of leadership qualities, including followership, which involves offering expertise in a supportive capacity without holding the official position of team leader. Desirable attributes of an effective follower may encompass actively listening to and valuing the viewpoints of others, exhibiting dedication, manifesting allegiance, and collaborating harmoniously with others to reach a consensus [50].

3.4.1.5 Domain of Program Management
Nurses must possess extensive knowledge of IPC and demonstrate proficiency in managing budgets, resources, staff, and programs with effectiveness and efficiency. By exhibiting proficient management and leadership abilities, nurses will bolster their reputation, exert greater influence, and secure a position of influence in important stakeholder discussions, guaranteeing that their IPC knowledge and viewpoint are represented in crucial decision-making processes. The crucial factor is achieving desired performance results, adjusting as necessary to continually minimize discrepancies between objectives and actual outcomes. An IPC nurse director and/or manager must possess additional competencies to effectively recruit, interview, onboard, coach, and foster the growth of talent within interdisciplinary teams [50].

3.4.1.6 Domain of Mentorship
The effectiveness of IPC nurses, particularly those who are new to the profession, can be greatly influenced by effective and timely mentorship. This is because IPC nurses come from diverse backgrounds within nursing and nonclinical disciplines and may not have had standardized training in infection prevention and control. Furthermore, the emphasis on executing and spreading preventive measures and interventions necessitates that IPC nurses acquire knowledge from one another's experiences. Skilled mentors share their infection prevention expertise by drawing on their professional backgrounds and helping colleagues apply theoretical principles and evidence-based guidelines to practical clinical settings [50].

3.4.1.7 Domain of Accountability
To maintain accountability for evidence-based practices, IPC nurses need to effectively operate within an organization. This is particularly important for activities that affect quality metrics, which are closely monitored by payers and regulators, and to prevent harm to patients. To uphold this standard of responsibility, IPC nurses must possess expertise in communication, education, relationship management, behavior modification, and facilitation. This is necessary to ensure that adherence to guidelines is created and that nurses are adequately trained and feel a sense of responsibility in preventing and controlling infections [50].

3.4.1.8 Domain of the Continuum of Care

The Continuum of Care subdomain encompasses the delivery of care across various health services, levels, and degrees of intensity. IPC standards cover a wide range of practice contexts, including acute care, behavioral health, long-term care, outpatient facilities, rehabilitation centers, community health centers, home care, and dialysis. IPC nurses should consider the IPC processes and products employed in each practice environment. They should also be aware of how they may affect the patient, their family, and the healthcare personnel as the patient transitions between different settings [50].

3.4.1.9 Advocacy Domain

To advance their positions of authority and responsibility, IPC nurses must actively promote and support IPC both at the individual facility level and on a broader national scale. At the national level, IPC nurses must stay updated on the political and regulatory healthcare environment. They should advocate for the profession and emphasize the crucial role that IPC plays in all levels of care, including regional, state, and local. IPC nurses should also educate policymakers and regulatory agencies about evidence-based IPC practices that safeguard patients, staff, and specific populations from infections. At the institutional level, IPC nurses must utilize their authority and sway to champion both the envisioned future and practical, gradual modifications that address the requirements of patients, visitors, staff, and the IPC program [50].

3.4.1.10 Competency Domain

Quality improvement is an essential foundation that IPC nurses must employ to systematically enhance care and decrease infections. Effective quality improvement necessitates thorough analysis and utilization of data, a comprehensive understanding of risk assessment, implementation of risk reduction strategies, and integration of performance improvement techniques, as well as a steadfast commitment to patient safety [50].

3.4.1.11 Domain of Data Utilization

To maintain and expand their impact, IPC nurses must be recognized as highly proficient users of data. Data use serves the objective of facilitating decision-making and goal-setting processes, as well as generating yearly plans and identifying priority improvement opportunities. It also involves soliciting participation from frontline personnel and providing information to leadership. The effective usage of data showcases the worth of the information accessible to the practitioner or the facility. In healthcare settings, information is obtained from both individuals and collectives [50].

3.4.1.12 Domain of Detection and Management of Outbreaks

An essential aspect of an IPC nurse's role is to continuously monitor and identify adverse occurrences, such as infections, that occur at a higher incidence than expected or include uncommon pathogens or adverse events. The essential elements for detecting and managing an outbreak consist of verifying the occurrence of the outbreak, informing relevant parties about the investigation, conducting a thorough examination of existing literature, establishing and improving the criteria for identifying cases and the methodology for finding them, creating a list of cases and a graph illustrating the epidemic's progression, observing and evaluating the activities related to the suspected source of the outbreak, collecting samples from the environment and devices if necessary, implementing and continuously evaluating control measures and their effectiveness, and conducting a detailed study of the outbreak if required [50].

3.4.1.13 Domain of Antimicrobial Stewardship

In the facility's antimicrobial stewardship activities, IPC nurses contribute their advisory experience and serve as leaders and advocates in this crucial area that has a growing impact on the health and safety of patients globally. IPC nurses play an active role in antimicrobial stewardship by identifying and detecting multidrug-resistant organisms in the population they serve. They help in the early detection of organisms and infected patients, ensure adherence to standard and transmission-based precautions, and implement infection prevention strategies like care bundle practices and hand hygiene. IPC nurses also develop and deliver educational programs for staff, patients, and visitors [50].

3.4.1.14 Domain of Research Competency

Research is a crucial and indispensable skill set that provides support and promotes progress in the IPC sector. This domain emphasizes the significance of applied research and implementation science. By integrating research structures into their position, the IPC nurse can effectively combine, utilize, and assess research data to develop and showcase their competence [50].

Implementation and dissemination science refers to a study that generates novel insights on the most effective methods for designing, implementing, and assessing quality improvement programs. An essential aspect of IPC nurses is their capacity to facilitate the integration of evidence-based practice and research findings into everyday practice. Implementing evidence-based practices in the field of IPC can be a challenging endeavor, and it should be noted that simply providing individuals with information does not guarantee a subsequent modification in their practices or behaviors. Mastery of implementation science equips one with the ability to determine the content and way guidelines and standards should influence daily clinical practice. It also enables them to incorporate evidence into accepted practice and implement it at the patient's bedside. Furthermore, it allows them to apply research published in scientific, peer-reviewed journals to policies and practices. IPC nurses in all settings should be knowledgeable of and utilize standardized frameworks to effectively incorporate evidence into practice. When assessing or planning an implementation study or activity, it is important to consider these frameworks. Dissemination science pertains to the deliberate and focused delivery of information and intervention items to a particular audience. Understanding the concepts of dissemination science immediately enhances the ability to educate and communicate effectively. Implementation involves utilizing ways to effectively incorporate evidence-based health interventions and modify practice patterns within specific settings, rather than only aiming to raise awareness [50].

3.5   Conclusion

It is crucial to acknowledge that quality improvement and research may appear identical, but they possess distinct characteristics. The purpose of research is to generate universal knowledge that can be used by others, while a quality improvement project within a facility aims to identify effective practices specific to that context without intending to influence the broader field. While it is not obligatory for all IPC nurses to design research studies, they do have a duty to contribute to the body of evidence by publishing their facility's work. Individuals without independent research capabilities might contribute to research studies by recognizing areas of knowledge that need further investigation and establishing research goals for their institutions. IPC nurses with extensive experience and knowledge are well-equipped to excel and make a significant impact in leading and engaging in local quality improvement programs [50].

References

1. Boyce J, Pittet D. HICPAC SHEA APIC IDSA hand hygiene task force: guideline for hand hygiene in health-care settings. Recommendations of the Healthcare Infection Control Practices Advisory Committee and the HICPAC. MMWR Recomm Rep. 2002;51(RR-16):1–44.
2. Croke L. Guideline for transmission-based precautions. AORN J. 2018;108(6):P7–9.
3. The European Operating Room Nurses Association (EORNA). EORNA Best Practice for perioperative care. Available at https://www.eorna.eu/wp-content/uploads/2020/09/EORNA-Best-Practice-for-Perioperative-Care-Edition-2020.pdf; 2020.
4. Link T. Guideline implementation: transmission-based precautions. AORN J. 2019;110(6):637–49.
5. Siegel JD, Rhinehart E, Jackson M, Chiarello L, Committee HICPA. Guideline for isolation precautions: preventing transmission of infectious agents in health care settings; 2007.
6. Kuhar DT, Carrico RM, Cox K, de Perio MA, Irwin KL, Lundstrom T, et al. Infection control in healthcare personnel: infrastructure and routine practices for occupational infection prevention and control services; 2019.
7. Organization WH. Global patient safety action plan 2021–2030: towards eliminating avoidable harm in health care. World Health Organization; 2021.
8. Ammouri AA, Tailakh AK, Muliira JK, Geethakrishnan R, Al KS. Patient safety culture among nurses. Int Nurs Rev. 2015;62(1):102–10.
9. Joint Commision, JC International. WHO Collaborating Center for Patient Safety's nine life-saving patient safety solutions. Jt Comm J Qual Patient Saf. 2007;33(7):427–62.
10. Lin F, Gillespie BM, Chaboyer W, Li Y, Whitelock K, Morley N, et al. Preventing surgical site infections: facilitators and barriers to nurses' adherence to clinical practice guidelines—a qualitative study. J Clin Nurs. 2019;28(9–10):1643–52.
11. Sermeus W. Understanding the role of nurses in patient safety: from evidence to policy with RN4CAST. BMC Nurs 2016;15.

12. Kakkar SK, Bala M, Arora V. Educating nursing staff regarding infection control practices and assessing its impact on the incidence of hospital-acquired infections. J Educ Health Promot. 2021;10(1):40.
13. Henneman EA. Recognizing the ordinary as extraordinary: insight into the "way we work" to improve patient safety outcomes. Am J Crit Care. 2017;26(4):272–7.
14. Vaismoradi M, Jordan S, Kangasniemi M. Patient participation in patient safety and nursing input–a systematic review. J Clin Nurs. 2015;24(5–6):627–39.
15. Vaismoradi M, Tella S, Logan P, Khakurel J, Vizcaya-Moreno F. Nurses' adherence to patient safety principles: a systematic review. Int J Environ Res Public Health. 2020;17(6):2028.
16. Machitidze M, Gogashvili M, Durglishvili N. The nurses' role in patient safety-literature review. Am J Biomed Sci Res. 2023;18(6):612–6.
17. Rashvand F, Ebadi A, Vaismoradi M, Salsali M, Yekaninejad MS, Griffiths P, et al. The assessment of safe nursing care: development and psychometric evaluation. J Nurs Manag. 2017;25(1):22–36.
18. Stewart A, Burton E, White J, Salmon M, Mcclelland A. Health for all nursing, global health and universal health coverage, vol. 3. The International Council of Nurses; 2019. p. 2021.
19. Ibrahim YS, Said A, Hamdy GK. Assessment of infection control practices in the neonatal intensive care unit. Egypt J Commun Med. 2011;29(4):27–45.
20. Frello AT, Carraro TE. Florence Nightingale's contributions: an integrative review of the literature. Escola Anna Nery. 2013;17:573–9.
21. Kilpatrick C, Tartari E, Gayet-Ageron A, Storr J, Tomczyk S, Allegranzi B, et al. Global hand hygiene improvement progress: two surveys using the WHO hand hygiene self-assessment framework. J Hosp Infect. 2018;100(2):202–6.
22. Belal S, Ahmed S, Elmosaad M, Mohamed Y, Abobaker R, Llaguno BB, Mohammed Sanad H, et al. In-services education program for improving nurses' performance regarding infection control measures in a rural hospital. Egypt J Health Care. 2020;11(2):702–18.
23. Benson S, Powers J. Your role in infection prevention. Nursing Made Incredibly Easy. 2011;9(3):36–41.
24. World Health Organisation. Improving infection prevention and control at the health facility: interim practical manual supporting implementation of the WHO guidelines on core components of infection prevention and control programmes. World Health Organization; 2018.
25. Oliveira A, Gama C, Paula A. Multimodal strategy to improve the adherence to hand hygiene and self-assessment of the institution for the promotion and practice of hand hygiene. J Public Health. 2018;40(1):163–8.
26. Sands K, Blanchard J, Grubbs K, Fredrick ON, Schlosser M, Korwek K, et al. Universal protection: operationalizing infection prevention guidance in the COVID-19 era. Jt Comm J Qual Patient Saf. 2021;47(5):327–32.
27. Chakravarthy M, Myatra SN, Rosenthal VD, Udwadia F, Gokul B, Divatia J, et al. The impact of the international nosocomial infection control consortium (INICC) multicenter, multidimensional hand hygiene approach in two cities of India. J Infect Public Health. 2015;8(2):177–86.
28. Allegranzi B, Gayet-Ageron A, Damani N, Bengaly L, McLaws M-L, Moro M-L, et al. Global implementation of WHO's multimodal strategy for improvement of hand hygiene: a quasi-experimental study. Lancet Infect Dis. 2013;13(10):843–51.
29. Khan HA, Baig FK, Mehboob R. Nosocomial infections: epidemiology, prevention, control and surveillance. Asian Pac J Trop Biomed. 2017;7(5):478–82.
30. Siahaan M, Handiyani H, Nurdiana N. Optimization of the roles and responsibilities of infection prevention and control nurse in hospital. Int J Nurs Health Serv (IJNHS). 2019;2(4):292–306.
31. Erasmus V, Daha TJ, Brug H, Richardus JH, Behrendt MD, Vos MC, et al. Systematic review of studies on compliance with hand hygiene guidelines in hospital care. Infect Control Hosp Epidemiol. 2010;31(3):283–94.
32. Mitchell BG, Gardner A, Stone PW, Hall L, Pogorzelska-Maziarz M. Hospital staffing and health care–associated infections: a systematic review of the literature. Jt Comm J Qual Patient Saf. 2018;44(10):613–22.

33. Gregory ME, MacEwan SR, Sova LN, Gaughan AA, Scheck MAA. A qualitative examination of interprofessional teamwork for infection prevention: development of a model and solutions. Med Care Res Rev. 2023;80(1):30–42.
34. Lalithabai DS, Hababeh MO, Wani TA, Aboshaiqah AE. Knowledge, attitude and beliefs of nurses regarding antibiotic use and prevention of antibiotic resistance. SAGE Open Nurs. 2022;8:23779608221076821.
35. Anwar M, Raziq A, Shoaib M, Baloch NS, Raza S, Sajjad B, et al. Exploring nurses' perception of antibiotic use and resistance: a qualitative inquiry. J Multidiscip Healthc. 2021;14:1599–608.
36. Thakur H, Rao R. Emphasis of infection prevention and control: a review. J Popul Therap Clin Pharmacol. 2024;31:2238–49.
37. Sharif A, Arbabisarjou A, Balouchi A, Ahmadidarrehsima S, Kashani HH. Knowledge, attitude, and performance of nurses toward hand hygiene in hospitals. Global J Health Sci. 2016;8(8):57.
38. Abdullah MI, Huang D, Sarfraz M, Ivascu L, Riaz A. Effects of internal service quality on nurses' job satisfaction, commitment and performance: mediating role of employee well-being. Nurs Open. 2021;8(2):607–19.
39. Purwanto A. The role of job satisfaction in the relationship between transformational leadership, knowledge management, work environment and performance. Solid State Technol. 2020;63(2s):293–314.
40. Saleem M, Khan Z. Healthcare simulation: an effective way of learning in health care. Pak J Med Sci. 2023;39(4):1185.
41. Koukourikos K, Tsaloglidou A, Kourkouta L, Papathanasiou IV, Iliadis C, Fratzana A, et al. Simulation in clinical nursing education. Acta Inform Med. 2021;29(1):15.
42. Mahdavi Ardestani SF, Adibi S, Golshan A, Sadeghian P. Factors influencing the effectiveness of E-learning in healthcare: a fuzzy ANP study. Healthcare. 2023.: MDPI;11(14):2035.
43. Carrico RM, Garrett H, Balcom D, Glowicz JB. Infection prevention and control core practices: a roadmap for nursing practice. Nursing 2023. 2018;48(8):22–8.
44. Kubde D, Badge AK, Ugemuge S, Shahu S. Importance of hospital infection control. Cureus. 2023;15(12):e50931.
45. Loveday HP, Wilson JA, Pratt RJ, Golsorkhi M, Tingle A, Bak A, et al. epic3: national evidence-based guidelines for preventing healthcare-associated infections in NHS hospitals in England. J Hosp Infect. 2014;86:S1–S70.
46. Storr J, Twyman A, Zingg W, Damani N, Kilpatrick C, Reilly J, et al. Core components for effective infection prevention and control programmes: new WHO evidence-based recommendations. Antimicrob Resist Infect Control. 2017;6:1–18.
47. Pittet D, Allegranzi B, Sax H, Dharan S, Pessoa-Silva CL, Donaldson L, et al. Evidence-based model for hand transmission during patient care and the role of improved practices. Lancet Infect Dis. 2006;6(10):641–52.
48. Haque M, McKimm J, Sartelli M, Dhingra S, Labricciosa FM, Islam S, et al. Strategies to prevent healthcare-associated infections: a narrative overview. Risk Manag Healthc Pol. 2020;13:1765–80.
49. Peters A, Otter J, Moldovan A, Parneix P, Voss A, Pittet D. Keeping hospitals clean and safe without breaking the bank; summary of the Healthcare Cleaning Forum 2018. Springer; 2018.
50. Billings C, Bernard H, Caffery L, Dolan SA, Donaldson J, Kalp E, et al. Advancing the profession: an updated future-oriented competency model for professional development in infection prevention and control. Am J Infect Control. 2019;47(6):602–14.
51. Bubb TN, Billings C, Berriel-Cass D, Bridges W, Caffery L, Cox J, et al. APIC professional and practice standards. Am J Infect Control. 2016;44(7):745–9.

European Union Directives and Guidelines

4

Tihana Gašpert

4.1 Introduction

In the current globalized world, infection control has become a critical concern that transcends national boundaries, as healthcare systems and patient populations are increasingly interconnected. In recognition of the significance of coordinated efforts in managing public health hazards, the European Union (EU) has implemented a comprehensive framework of directives and guidelines designed to improve infection prevention and control in all member states. These regulations are intended to facilitate the harmonization of policies and practices across various countries and guarantee a high standard of patient safety and care.

Nurses are essential to the successful implementation of these EU directives, as they are the primary guardians of patient health. In addition to adhering to infection prevention protocols, they are accountable for educating patients, training healthcare personnel, and contributing to the development of national and local strategies. The commitment and expertise of nurses are crucial in the fight against healthcare-associated infections (HAIs), as the effective adaptation and integration of EU regulations into national healthcare systems are contingent upon their hands-on involvement.

Infection prevention and control (IPC) within healthcare settings are addressed by numerous directives and regulations of the European Union (EU). These directives are a component of the overarching EU strategy to uphold high standards of public health in all member states, reduce healthcare-associated infections (HAIs), and assure patient safety.

T. Gašpert (✉)
University Hospital Rijeka, Rijeka, Croatia

Faculty of Health Sciences, University of Maribor, Maribor, Slovenia

35

4.2   Directives

Healthcare professionals must comprehend the impact of EU directives on infection prevention management and how they are adapted and implemented at the national level in this context. This knowledge not only improves the efficacy of nurses in fulfilling their responsibilities but also enables them to contribute to the ongoing enhancement of infection control practices in the European healthcare sector.

4.2.1   Recommendation of the Council on Patient Safety, Including the Prevention and Control of Healthcare-Associated Infections (2009/C 151/01)

Although this recommendation is not legally binding, it is essential in assisting EU member states in their efforts to enhance patient safety throughout the region. It underscores the necessity of formulating comprehensive national strategies that are designed to mitigate healthcare-associated infections (HAIs). The recommendation promotes the training of healthcare personnel to ensure adherence to best practices in infection control and the establishment of surveillance systems to monitor infection rates. Furthermore, it promotes the establishment of systems that facilitate the reporting and learning from adverse events, such as HAIs, to cultivate a culture of continuous improvement in healthcare environments.

Patient safety and healthcare-associated infections (HAIs) within the European Union (EU) are significant public health concerns, as underscored by the Council Recommendation on Patient Safety, which encompasses the prevention and control of healthcare-associated infections. The recommendation establishes a framework for EU member states to enhance patient safety, acknowledging the estimated 8–12% of patients who experience adverse events during healthcare and the 4.1 million cases of HAIs that result in 37,000 fatalities annually.

The necessity of comprehensive national policies and programs that prioritize patient safety and integrate it into healthcare practices at all levels is underscored by the recommendation. It promotes the development of secure healthcare systems, patient empowerment, and the involvement of health professional organizations using information and communication technologies.

Additionally, the recommendation promotes the development of nonpunitive reporting and learning systems to identify and resolve adverse events, the enhancement of patient safety education and training for healthcare professionals, and the collection of comparable data across the EU to assess and enhance patient safety outcomes.

The recommendation encourages member states to develop and execute national strategies that are designed to prevent and manage HAIs. This encompasses the improvement of patient information regarding HAIs, the development of infection prevention and control measures, the enhancement of surveillance systems, and the promotion of specialized training for healthcare personnel.

Essentially, the objective of this recommendation is to establish a coordinated and comprehensive strategy throughout the EU to enhance patient safety and decrease the incidence of healthcare-associated infections. This will be achieved through the implementation of targeted strategies, education, surveillance, and policy development [1].

4.2.2   Directive 2011/24/EU on Patients' Rights in Cross-Border Healthcare

The European Parliament and the Council's Directive 2011/24/EU, which was adopted on 9 March 2011, set the framework for patients' rights to access healthcare services in all EU member states. Up to the amount that would have been covered if the treatment had been received at home, patients are permitted to seek medical treatment in any EU country and receive reimbursement from their home country's healthcare system under the directive. This provision guarantees that patients in the EU can receive safe and high-quality healthcare, while simultaneously preserving the financial obligations of their respective national healthcare systems.

The directive underscores the significance of quality and safety standards, mandating that healthcare providers in the EU adhere to their respective national regulations. These standards are also entitled to be disclosed to patients in order to assist them in making well-informed decisions about their treatment options. The directive establishes National Contact Points in each member state to facilitate this process. These points are responsible for providing patients with comprehensive information about their rights, available healthcare services, and the quality and safety of treatments they may receive abroad.

Furthermore, the directive guarantees that prescriptions issued in one member state are recognized in others, thereby enabling patients to continue their treatment seamlessly across borders. It also promotes collaboration among national healthcare systems, such as the exchange of information, mutual recognition of medical qualifications, and collaboration on eHealth initiatives [2].

This directive is essential in guaranteeing that patients in the EU have the right to access healthcare services across member states, with the potential for reimbursement for treatments received abroad under specific circumstances. It also requires healthcare providers to adhere to high standards of care, which inherently encompasses implementing effective infection prevention measures. The directive mandates that member states exchange information regarding healthcare providers to guarantee transparency and confidence in the quality and safety of cross-border healthcare services. This is essential for preventing infection, as it guarantees that patients who receive care outside of their country of origin are safeguarded by the same stringent standards enforced domestically.

4.2.3   Directive 2000/54/EC on the Protection of Workers from Risks Related to Exposure to Biological Agents at Work

The objective of this directive is to protect healthcare workers and other employees from the hazards that are linked to exposure to biological agents, including pathogens that can cause infections. It necessitates that employers identify and evaluate these hazards in the workplace and implement strategies to prevent or reduce exposure. These measures encompass the provision of personal protective equipment (PPE), the implementation of vaccination programs, and the enforcement of appropriate hygiene practices. Additionally, the directive requires that workers be provided with sufficient training and information regarding the protective measures in place and the potential risks involved, thereby enabling them to effectively safeguard themselves.

The protection of workers from the risks associated with exposure to biological agents in the workplace is the subject of Directive 2000/54/EC of the European Parliament and of the Council, which was implemented on 18 September 2000. This directive is essential for occupations that are susceptible to the transmission of infectious diseases by microorganisms, including bacteria, viruses, fungi, and other biological entities. The directive establishes a comprehensive framework that is designed to mitigate and manage these risks to guarantee the health and safety of workers.

The directive's fundamental requirement is for employers to implement a comprehensive risk assessment to identify potential biological agent hazards. This evaluation must consider the nature of the work being performed, the biological agents that workers may encounter, and the potential health consequences of such exposure. Employers are required to implement suitable preventive and protective measures to mitigate the identified risks by the results of this assessment.

The directive categorizes biological agents into four distinct risk categories, each of which poses a varying degree of risk to human health. From agents that are unlikely to cause disease (Group 1) to those that cause severe disease, present a serious hazard to workers, and pose a significant risk of disseminating to the community, with no effective treatment available (Group 4), the classification ranges. The necessary safety measures become increasingly stringent as the risk level increases, particularly for agents classified in Groups 3 and 4. When necessary, employers must implement advanced control measures, including vaccination, personal protective equipment (PPE), and containment facilities, for higher-risk agents.

The directive requires employers to furnish workers with adequate information, instruction, and training regarding the hazards of exposure to biological agents and the necessary precautions to be taken, in addition to instituting safety measures. Workers must be apprised of the results of the risk assessment, the health hazards that are associated with it, and the protective measures that have been implemented. The directive also mandates that workers who are exposed to biological agents undergo routine health surveillance to facilitate the early identification of any adverse health effects.

The directive specifies the classification of biological agents, the reporting of incidents involving exposure, and the maintenance of records related to workers' exposure and health surveillance. The objective of this framework is to establish a secure work environment by guaranteeing that all requisite measures are implemented to safeguard employees from biological hazards, thereby reducing the incidence of work-related infections and diseases [3].

Directive 2000/54/EC has been subject to numerous amendments since its adoption, with the most recent consolidated version being dated 24 June 2020. The directive has been updated to incorporate new scientific knowledge, technological advancements, and changes in workplace risks. This has ensured that the directive remains relevant and effective in protecting workers from biological hazards in an ever-evolving work environment.

4.2.4   Regulation (EU) 2017/745 on Medical Devices and Regulation (EU) 2017/746 on In Vitro Diagnostic Medical Devices

These regulations are essential for guaranteeing that medical devices and diagnostic instruments utilized in healthcare facilities throughout the European Union adhere to rigorous safety and performance standards. To prevent infections that may result from their use, it is imperative that these devices are designed, produced, and monitored post-market. The regulations specify precise standards for the sterilization, disinfection, and management of medical devices to guarantee their safety and absence of contamination for patient use. These regulations make a substantial contribution to the overarching objective of infection prevention in healthcare environments by establishing rigorous standards for medical devices [4].

Regulation (EU) 2017/745 concentrates on medical devices, which encompass a diverse array of products, including surgical instruments, implants, and medical software. It establishes more stringent standards for the certification and monitoring of these devices. The regulation promotes transparency by mandating the establishment of a European database on medical devices (EUDAMED), which provides access to information regarding devices, manufacturers, and clinical investigations. It also enhances the traceability of devices throughout their lifecycle and post-market surveillance [5].

In vitro diagnostic medical devices, which are utilized to conduct tests on samples, such as blood or tissue, to diagnose diseases or conditions, are regulated by Regulation (EU) 2017/746. This regulation implements a classification system that is risk-based, with more stringent controls for devices that pose a greater risk. It also underscores the necessity of robust clinical evidence to substantiate the safety and functionality of these devices [6].

Both regulations impose a greater burden on manufacturers to guarantee the safety and efficacy of their products. The manufacturers are obligated to maintain detailed technical documentation, conduct rigorous clinical evaluations, and implement quality management systems. Furthermore, the regulations strengthen the function of notified bodies, which are autonomous organizations that are responsible for evaluating the compliance of devices with EU regulations.

These regulations represent a substantial change in the regulation of medical devices and in vitro diagnostic devices in the EU, to enhance patient safety, establish more consistent and transparent regulatory requirements, and promoting innovation in the healthcare sector. They replace the previous directives in these areas, providing a more coherent and robust regulatory framework [4].

4.3   EU Guidelines on the Prudent Use of Antimicrobials in Human Health

These guidelines are a component of the European Union's initiative to address antimicrobial resistance (AMR), a significant public health challenge that is closely associated with infection prevention. They encourage healthcare professionals to prescribe antibiotics only when necessary and in a responsible manner, thereby promoting the responsible use of antibiotics in human medicine. The guidelines also underscore the significance of infection prevention and control practices that mitigate the necessity for antibiotics, including vaccination, effective hand hygiene, and the implementation of aseptic techniques. These guidelines contribute to the prevention of the spread of resistant bacteria and the preservation of the efficacy of current treatments by reducing the use of superfluous antibiotics [7].

The guidelines underscore the significance of employing antimicrobials sparingly and only when they are unquestionably necessary. This entails the restriction of antimicrobial prescriptions and administration to bacterial infections that have been confirmed or are highly suspected. If antimicrobials are ineffective in treating viral infections, alternative treatments or supportive care should be considered.

The guidelines underscore the importance of proper antimicrobial stewardship. This entails the selection of the most suitable antimicrobial agent by the specific pathogen and its resistance profile, as well as the assurance that the dosage and duration of treatment are sufficient to effectively eradicate the infection without fostering resistance.

The guidelines also emphasize the necessity of conducting comprehensive diagnostic procedures before the commencement of treatment to prevent the superfluous use of antimicrobials. Healthcare professionals are encouraged to remain informed about the most recent evidence and recommendations for antimicrobial use, as well as to discuss the significance of adhering to prescribed treatments with patients [7].

4.4   EU Framework for Action on Antimicrobial Resistance (AMR)

This framework offers a comprehensive strategy for confronting antimicrobial resistance, a burgeoning issue in infection control. It encompasses measures that are essential to the prevention of infections and the reduction of the dissemination of resistant bacteria, which are essential components of infection prevention initiatives. Enhanced surveillance of antimicrobial resistance and use is emphasized in the framework at both the national and EU levels. It also advocates for the enhancement of infection prevention and control measures, including the promotion of the development of novel diagnostic tools and treatments and the enhancement of hygiene practices in healthcare settings. The objective of this coordinated strategy is to safeguard public health by decreasing the prevalence of resistant infections throughout the European Union [8].

The report emphasizes that AMR poses a substantial threat to global health, potentially resulting in a situation in which prevalent infections are rendered untreatable. This could lead to increased morbidity and mortality rates, which could place a burden on healthcare systems worldwide. In terms of economics, the report predicts that the failure to address AMR could result in substantial financial losses because of increased healthcare costs and decreased productivity.

The review provides several suggestions for addressing AMR, such as expanding the research and development of novel antibiotics and alternatives, enhancing infection prevention and control measures, and improving the stewardship of antimicrobial drugs. It underscores the necessity of a global, coordinated strategy that involves the pharmaceutical industry, governments, healthcare providers, and the public to effectively address this crisis.

The review outlines the critical role that nurses play in confronting antimicrobial resistance. They are essential for the successful implementation of effective antimicrobial stewardship and infection prevention strategies, as they are on the front lines of patient care. Initially, the role of nurses in antimicrobial stewardship is indispensable. They are required to comply with the guidelines for prescribing and administering antimicrobials, ensuring that they are only used when necessary and appropriate. Nurses are responsible for monitoring patient responses to treatment, which assists in the formulation of informed decisions regarding the continuation, modification, or discontinuation of antimicrobial therapies. Secondly, AMR is directly influenced by the fundamental aspect of nursing practice, which is infection prevention and control. To prevent the transmission of infections, nurses must adhere to strict infection control protocols, including the use of personal protective equipment (PPE), sterile techniques, and hand hygiene. Minimizing the risk of resistance is achieved through the implementation of effective infection control, which reduces the necessity for antimicrobials.

Furthermore, nurses are accountable for instructing patients regarding the appropriate utilization of antimicrobials. This entails elucidating the significance of adhering to prescribed medication regimens, the potential repercussions of nonadherence, and the hazards of misuse. Proper patient education is essential for the effective use of antimicrobials and the prevention of resistance. In addition, nurses are essential in the processes of monitoring and reporting. They document and observe patient outcomes, and any adverse effects associated with antimicrobial treatments. It is essential to report these observations to identify trends in resistance and modify treatment protocols as necessary.

Lastly, it is essential to work in conjunction with other healthcare professionals. To guarantee that antimicrobial prescriptions are consistent with the most effective practices and guidelines, nurses collaborate with physicians, pharmacists, and other healthcare professionals. This collaborative approach promotes effective stewardship and improves the overall quality of patient care [8].

4.5 European Centre for Disease Prevention and Control (ECDC) Guidelines

The ECDC is essential in providing EU member states with technical reports and guidelines that enhance infection prevention and control practices. Although these guidelines are not legally binding, they have a significant impact on the development of national policies and strategies. The ECDC offers advice on a diverse array of topics, including the use of personal protective equipment (PPE), hand hygiene, and outbreak management. It also provides best practices for managing specific infections, such as *Clostridium difficile* and MRSA, which are common challenges in healthcare contexts. The ECDC ensures a high standard of patient safety and care throughout the region by disseminating evidence-based recommendations, which serve to harmonize infection prevention efforts across Europe [9].

4.6 Council Recommendation on Stepping Up EU Actions to Combat Antimicrobial Resistance in a One Health Approach 2023/C 220/01

The 2023 Council Recommendation on "Stepping Up EU Actions to Combat Antimicrobial Resistance in a One Health Approach" underscores the importance of a comprehensive framework that integrates human, animal, and environmental health to implement a coordinated strategy to address antimicrobial resistance (AMR). The document emphasizes the necessity of improved surveillance systems that monitor the use and resistance of antimicrobials in these interconnected domains. The objective of this method is to facilitate a more comprehensive comprehension of AMR and to inform more effective interventions.

The recommendation urges the enhancement of antimicrobial stewardship programs in a variety of sectors, such as agriculture, veterinary practices, and healthcare. This entails the promotion of responsible antimicrobial use and the implementation of practices that reduce the risk of resistance. The objective is to mitigate the dissemination of resistant bacteria by enhancing hygiene and control practices in healthcare settings, agriculture, and other pertinent environments. Additionally, enhanced infection prevention and control measures are being prioritized.

Furthermore, the recommendation emphasizes the significance of investing in research and innovation. This encompasses the promotion of the development of novel antimicrobials, vaccines, and alternative treatments, as well as the investigation of innovative methods to prevent and control infections. Public awareness and education are also critical components, to promote the safe and effective use of antimicrobials and foster a greater understanding of AMR among the public.

4.7   Conclusion

Collectively, these directives and guidelines establish a comprehensive framework for infection prevention in the European Union. They guarantee that healthcare systems in all member states comply with stringent patient safety standards and are adequately prepared to address the obstacles presented by antimicrobial resistance and healthcare-associated infections. The EU's objective is to safeguard public health and guarantee the safety of healthcare personnel and patients using these coordinated endeavors [10].

Literature

1. Simerka P. Council Recommendation of 9 June 2009 on patient safety, including the prevention and control of healthcare associated infections. Off J Eur Union. 2009:1–6.
2. Union E. Directive 2011/24/EU of the European Parliament and of the Council of 9 March 2011 on the application of patients' rights in cross-border healthcare. Off J Eur Union. 2011;
3. Darmoris O. Legal regulation of workers' health and safety working with biological agents in the European Union. Evropský politický a právní diskurz. 2017;2:125–9.
4. Barnard C, Peers S. European union law. Oxford University Press; 2023.
5. Annex I. Regulation (EU) 2017/745 Annexes. Regulation (EU); 2017:745.
6. Kahles A, Goldschmid H, Volckmar A-L, Ploeger C, Kazdal D, Penzel R, et al. Regulation (EU) 2017/746 (IVDR): practical implementation of annex I in pathology. Die Pathologie. 2023;44(Suppl 2):86–95.
7. Commission E. EU Guidelines for the prudent use of antimicrobials in human health. Off J Eur Union. 2017;212:914–5.
8. O'neill J. Antimicrobial resistance: tackling a crisis for the health and wealth of nations. Rev Antimicrob Resist. 2014.
9. Zarb P, Coignard B, Griskeviciene J, Muller A, Vankerckhoven V, Weist K, et al. The European Centre for Disease Prevention and Control (ECDC) pilot point prevalence survey of healthcare-associated infections and antimicrobial use. Eurosurveillance. 2012;17(46):20316.
10. Jeschke J. Regulatory and scientific strategies to combat antimicrobial resistance in the EU. 2024.

Infection Prevention in Non-Conventional Environments

5

Silvana Gastaldi

5.1 Introduction

Currently, two billion people live in countries where development outcomes are affected by fragility, conflict, and violence (FCV). By 2030, nearly 60% of the global poor will live in such situations [1]. Conflict-affected and vulnerable settings encompass situations of crisis where people experience humanitarian emergencies, prolonged disruptions to critical public services, significant armed conflict, extreme adversity, or acute, protracted, or complex emergencies. The health service needs in these environments are substantial [2].

These settings face numerous constraints, including the breakdown of health systems, an inadequate workforce, lack of safety and security, including attacks on healthcare, and a scarcity of resources [2].

Infection prevention and control (IPC) is a cornerstone of effective and quality of healthcare delivery but implementing IPC measures in non conventional settings such as conflict zones, remote areas, and regions with inadequate infrastructure presents unique challenges [3]. This paragraph synthesizes insights and strategies from various studies and reports, focusing on how healthcare providers manage IPC in environments fraught with resource limitations, logistical constraints, and ongoing violence.

S. Gastaldi (✉)
Independent Researcher, Mazzano, Italy

5.2   Challenges in Nonconventional Environments

5.2.1   Limited Access to Resources

One of the primary challenges in infection control in conflict-ridden and vulnerable settings is the scarcity of resources [3]. Settings of extreme adversity, often lack adequate healthcare infrastructure, including sterile equipment, proper sanitation facilities, clean water, and trained personnel essential for implementing IPC measures [3]. These limitations hinder maintaining a hygienic environment. Additionally, the frequent power outages and water supply disruptions further complicate infection control efforts. The constant influx of patients, particularly those with traumatic injuries, continuously challenges Surgical Site Infection (SSI) prevention. The conflict situation in certain countries places additional strain on already limited resources because strikes and security issues hinder the delivery and collection of essential supplies, resulting in supply chain disruptions.

Research by Allegranzi et al. [4] highlights the burden of healthcare-associated infections (HAIs) in developing countries, where resource constraints are pronounced. In conflict settings, the situation is exacerbated by the diversion of resources to emergency medical care and security needs. As a result, healthcare facilities struggle to maintain basic infection prevention and control (IPC) measures, such as hand hygiene and environmental hygiene.

Addressing the challenge of limited resources requires innovative solutions tailored to conflict zones. For example, the World Health Organization (WHO) has developed trauma kits equipped with essential instruments and supplies for major trauma, optimizing the available equipment [5]. Muhrbeck et al. [6], in a retrospective study in International Committee of Red Cross (ICRC) hospitals, compared different trauma scores to predict resource consumption and in-hospital mortality in resource-scarce conflict settings. WHO also provides community guidance on alternative hand hygiene strategies when clean running water, soap, or alcohol-based hand rubs are unavailable, such as using sand or ash and self-produced hand sanitizers [7]. Training local healthcare workers in improvised sterilization techniques and waste management practices can further mitigate the impact of resource constraints on IPC and in particular on SSIs.

Ongoing conflict disrupts supply chains, leading to shortages of essential medical supplies like antibiotics, disinfectants, and surgical instruments. Nguyen D. et al. [8] examined the incidence and etiology of SSIs in Vietnam, highlighting how disrupted supply chains impact infection control efforts. The authors identified procurement delays of surgical supplies and medications as factors contributing to the high prevalence of SSIs in conflict-affected areas [8]. Furthermore, the quality of available supplies may be compromised due to substandard manufacturing, improper storage conditions, or reliance on local market purchases. Addressing supply chain disruptions and adapting IPC measures to the local context, such as creating ad hoc IPC guidelines like WHO did for Gaza [9], requires collaboration among healthcare providers and humanitarian organizations. Coordination should focus on ensuring timely access to essential medical supplies, establishing contingency plans, and strengthening local procurement and distribution networks. Innovative approaches and decentralized production of essential medications can also help mitigate the impact of supply chain disruptions on infection control. The availability of medical supplies, including personal protective equipment (PPE), is another critical issue. In many conflict settings, disrupted supply chains lead to shortages that hinder effective IPC. For instance, in Yemen, the protracted conflict has severely impacted the availability of medical supplies, compromising hygiene standards and infection prevention [10]. Additionally, the lack of trained healthcare personnel is a significant barrier. Many conflict zones experience high turnover rates among healthcare workers due to environmental dangers, instability, and staff evacuation. For this reason, training and retaining skilled healthcare workers who can implement and monitor IPC practices is challenging, as seen in conflict-affected regions like South Sudan and the Central African Republic [11].

5.2.2   Infrastructure Deficiencies

The absence of reliable electricity and refrigeration hampers the storage and administration of vaccines and medications. Maintaining cold chains for vaccines is particularly problematic in regions without stable electricity. Inadequate infrastructure also affects water supply and sanitation systems. Many health facilities in conflict zones lack running water, making it difficult to maintain hygiene standards necessary for IPC. The situation is further exacerbated by the damage to healthcare facilities caused by ongoing violence, which can render existing infrastructure unusable.

For instance, in Syria the destruction of healthcare infrastructure has led to significant challenges in maintaining IPC. Many hospitals and clinics have been damaged or destroyed, forcing healthcare providers to work in makeshift facilities that lack basic amenities such as clean water and proper waste disposal systems [12].

5.2.3   Humanitarian Crises

Natural disasters, disease outbreaks, and conflicts often displace large populations into makeshift settlements with poor sanitation and overcrowded conditions, which facilitate the rapid spread of infectious diseases. Médecins Sans Frontières (MSF) in Nigeria and Yemen refugee camps documented outbreaks of waterborne diseases due to poor sanitation [13].

Overcrowding in refugee camps, temporary shelters, or healthcare facilities creates environments where infectious diseases can spread rapidly as happening in high-risk settings. The close quarters and lack of adequate sanitation facilities mean that diseases such as cholera, typhoid, and respiratory infections are common. In the Rohingya refugee camps in Bangladesh, for example, the combination of overcrowding and inadequate sanitation has led to repeated outbreaks of COVID-19 disease [14].

5.3   Innovations and Strategies

5.3.1   Community-Based Approaches

Empowering local communities through education and training can significantly enhance IPC efforts. Community health workers trained in basic infection prevention practices have shown to reduce infection rates in rural Afghanistan [15].

Community engagement is critical in areas where healthcare access is limited. Training community health workers to deliver IPC education and basic healthcare services can bridge the gap. During the West Africa Ebola outbreak, community health workers played a pivotal role in educating the public about hygiene practices and reducing the spread of the virus [16].

Additionally, involving community leaders and local organizations in IPC initiatives can foster trust and encourage community-wide adherence to hygiene practices. In Sierra Leone, local leaders were instrumental in mobilizing communities to adopt IPC measures during the Ebola outbreak [17].

5.3.2   Technology Adaptations

Adapting technologies for low-resource settings is critical. For instance, solar-powered refrigerators for vaccine storage and portable water purification systems have been successfully implemented in conflict zones, improving healthcare delivery despite electricity shortages [18]. Innovations such as portable handwashing stations and mobile clinics equipped with essential IPC tools have proven effective in remote and conflict-affected areas. In the Democratic Republic of Congo, mobile clinics have been deployed to provide healthcare services, including IPC, to populations in hard-to-reach areas [19].

Moreover, telemedicine has emerged as a valuable tool in conflict settings, allowing healthcare providers to offer guidance and support remotely. This approach has been particularly beneficial during the COVID-19 pandemic, where travel restrictions and safety concerns limited in-person consultations [20].

5.3.3   Policy and Advocacy

The field of infection prevention and control (IPC) intersects clinical practice and public health, aiming to reduce infection risks for patients, health workers, and the wider community while combating antimicrobial resistance (AMR) [21].

IPC policies and practices, referred to as IPC programmes, are integral to healthcare safety, quality, global health security, and emergency health response [21]. These programmes are essential for achieving the United Nations Sustainable Development Goals (SDGs), as highlighted in the World Health Organization (WHO) Global Strategy on IPC [22].

However, IPC programmes can be resource-intensive, and their environmental impacts are only beginning to be understood [23, 24]. It is crucial for international organizations and governments to prioritize IPC in humanitarian aid policies and funding. Advocacy is needed to mobilize resources for sustainable healthcare infrastructure improvements, especially in low-resource or unconventional settings, such as countries affected by war.

Policy initiatives should focus on integrating IPC measures into all aspects of humanitarian aid and health service delivery. For instance, the Sphere Standards, which provide guidelines for humanitarian response, emphasize the importance of IPC in maintaining health and dignity in disaster-affected populations [25].

Emergency Medical Teams (EMTs), the EMT Initiative, and its global network are critical in this context. They focus on establishing common quality standards and recommendations for medical teams to rapidly and effectively respond to health emergencies. By strengthening and supporting national capacities through strong collaboration and coordination, the EMT initiative enables countries to access trusted partnerships for interoperable surge capacities and facilitates the deployment of their global network to deliver care when required. Integrating EMTs into IPC programmes like in the case of "Minimum standards and recommendations for medical teams responding to highly infectious disease outbreaks" [26], can enhance the efficiency and effectiveness of health emergency responses, ensuring that IPC measures are upheld even in the most challenging environments.

Advocacy efforts can also highlight the need for long-term investments in health infrastructure and workforce development. Building resilient health systems that can withstand crises is essential for sustaining IPC efforts. The Global Health Security Agenda is an example of a multinational initiative aimed at strengthening health systems to prevent and respond to infectious disease threats [27].

5.4 Overcoming Challenges Specific to Conflict Settings

5.4.1 Surgical Site Infections

Healthcare facilities in conflict zones face the dual challenge of providing urgent medical care to violence victims while mitigating the risk of SSIs. Limited resources, disrupted supply chains, and increased patient vulnerability exacerbate these challenges [4, 28]. As mentioned previously, strategies such as using trauma kits [5], improvised sterilization techniques, and alternative hand hygiene methods have been developed to address these issues [7].

Trauma care in conflict settings often involves complex surgical procedures with high risks of infection. The lack of sterile environments and the prevalence of MDROs complicate post-surgical care. In Iraq, for example, the high incidence of SSIs among war-injured patients highlights the need for stringent IPC protocols and the development of context-specific guidelines [29].

Furthermore, the training of healthcare workers in conflict settings to recognize and manage SSIs is crucial. Implementing standardized protocols and providing continuous education can help improve outcomes.

5.4.2   Disrupted Supply Chains

Conflict disrupts supply chains, leading to shortages of essential medical supplies. Collaborative efforts among healthcare providers, humanitarian organizations, and local authorities are essential to ensure timely access to necessary supplies [30]. Innovative solutions like 3D printing of surgical instruments have been explored to mitigate the impact of supply chain disruptions [31]. Establishing local production facilities for essential medical supplies can also reduce dependency on external supply chains. Greater resources should be allocated to researching the effects of conflicts on healthcare and exploring technological and innovative solutions to lessen the damage [32].

Coordination among international aid agencies and local governments is vital to manage supply chains effectively. Establishing centralized hubs for the distribution of medical supplies can ensure that resources are allocated efficiently. The Logistics Cluster, led by the World Food Programme, has been instrumental in coordinating supply chains in humanitarian crises [33].

5.4.3   Increased Patient Vulnerability

Conflict-affected populations are more vulnerable to infections due to malnutrition, overcrowded living conditions, and limited access to healthcare. Community engagement and health education programs focusing on hygiene practices and wound care are crucial in mitigating infection risks [34, 35].

Addressing the underlying factors that contribute to patient vulnerability, such as malnutrition and poor living conditions, is essential. Integrating IPC efforts with nutrition and shelter programs can enhance overall health outcomes. In Yemen, multi-sectoral approaches that combine health, nutrition, and WASH (water, sanitation, and hygiene) interventions have shown promise in reducing infection rates [36].

Additionally, targeted interventions for high-risk groups, such as pregnant women and children, are necessary. Providing maternal and child health services that include IPC measures can prevent infections and improve survival rates.

5.5   Direct Impacts of Conflict on IPC

Conflict introduces new wound patterns and complexities, such as those seen with injuries from improvised explosive devices (IEDs), which pose significant challenges for IPC. Understanding the bacteriology of war wounds is essential for effective management and infection prevention. For example, studies have shown shifts in microbial composition over time, highlighting the need for tailored IPC strategies [37].

War-related injuries often involve complex wound care that requires advanced IPC measures. The presence of foreign bodies and extensive tissue damage increases the risk of infection. Research in conflict zones like Afghanistan and Iraq has demonstrated the importance of early and aggressive debridement, appropriate antibiotic use, and meticulous wound care in preventing infections [38].

Furthermore, the psychological impact of conflict on both patients and healthcare providers can affect IPC practices. High-stress environments can lead to lapses in protocol adherence and increased risk of infections. Providing mental health support and stress management training for healthcare workers is essential for maintaining IPC standards.

5.6 Combating Multidrug-Resistant Organisms in Non-conventional Settings

The rise of MDROs in conflict zones is a growing concern. Effective IPC practices are imperative to prevent the spread of these organisms. Measures such as routine microbiological screenings, isolation units, and antimicrobial stewardship protocols have been implemented to address this issue [39, 40].

For example, the International Red Cross Committee (ICRC) response to Antimicrobial Stewardship (AMS) challenges in conflict settings has primarily focused on its hospital program. Through a qualitative study, ICRC established the foundation for an evidence-based approach to enhance IPC awareness, processes, and practices [35].

The spread of MDROs is facilitated by the frequent movement of populations and the use of broad-spectrum antibiotics in conflict settings. Implementing robust surveillance systems to monitor antibiotic resistance patterns is critical. This is why initiatives such as the Global Antimicrobial Resistance Surveillance System (GLASS) [41], which offers a framework for monitoring and addressing antimicrobial resistance, are crucial.

In addition to surveillance, promoting the rational use of antibiotics through stewardship programs can help curb the rise of MDROs. Training healthcare providers on appropriate prescribing practices and implementing guidelines for antibiotic use are key strategies. Médecins Sans Frontières (MSF) has developed a structured approach to implementing AMS in hospitals, including those in conflict-affected regions such as in the Middle East by featuring a dedicated IPC officer, SOPs for antibiotic prescription and administration, and comprehensive AMS implementation, including optimized antibiotic use and guidance based on susceptibility testing in high-quality labs [42].

This strategy incorporates standardized antibiotic treatment guidelines, context-adapted antibiotic forms, and the identification, training, and mentoring of antibiotic stewardship focal points. It also involves the adoption of both restrictive and persuasive stewardship strategies, regular point prevalence surveys of antibiotic prescriptions, and, whenever possible, access to diagnostic facilities with quality-assured microbiology laboratories [43].

Isolation and infection control measures in healthcare facilities must be strengthened to prevent the spread of MDROs. Designing facilities with dedicated isolation units and ensuring strict adherence to infection control protocols can mitigate transmission. The use of barrier nursing techniques and enhanced cleaning protocols in conflict zones like Syria has proven effective in controlling MDRO outbreaks [32].

5.7 Enhancing Surgical and General Healthcare Services in Conflict-Affected and Vulnerable Settings

In humanitarian trauma surgery projects, the incidence of SSI is higher, likely due in part to the substantial number of contaminated and neglected injuries from blasts, gunshot wounds, and road trauma [44, 45]. Notably, the use of external fixation devices in trauma surgery programs has improved recovery times for long bone fractures. However, SSIs in these patients, especially when caused by multidrug-resistant organisms, are particularly difficult and costly to manage. The relatively high SSI rates in poor and conflict-affected contexts may also stem from non-hospital factors, such as a higher proportion of patients with compromised immune systems, delays in seeking medical care, and post-discharge issues, including inadequate access to clean water and incomplete follow-up [28].

While surgical care in conflict zones often focuses on trauma, there is also a significant need for general surgical services, including obstetric emergencies and infectious diseases. Addressing these needs requires comprehensive IPC strategies that go beyond trauma care [46].

Obstetric care in conflict zones faces unique challenges, with high rates of maternal and neonatal infections due to inadequate facilities and lack of trained personnel. Implementing IPC measures in maternity wards and training birth attendants in hygiene practices can significantly reduce infection rates.

Populations in conflict areas face an increased risk of polio and other vaccine-preventable disease (VPD) outbreaks for several reasons [47]. Firstly, factors such as poor nutritional status, overcrowding, and unsanitary conditions in these settings create an environment conducive to VPD outbreaks [47]. Secondly, the destruction of healthcare infrastructure due to armed conflict compromises immunization and other routine health services, leading to a subpopulation of unimmunized or under-immunized individuals vulnerable to disease outbreaks [47]. Thirdly, when outbreaks occur in these settings, they spread rapidly and are likely to persist due to inadequate surveillance, lack of treatment facilities, insufficiently trained or unavailable health personnel, and challenges in outbreak response planning and implementation [47]. Lastly, forced displacements across national and international borders can lead to large outbreaks in other areas, often spread by asymptomatic individuals. These factors collectively result in a higher disease burden and mortality for this vulnerable population and contribute to the global spread of diseases [47].

The integration of IPC measures into routine healthcare services is essential for sustaining health gains. Training healthcare workers across all levels of care in IPC practices and ensuring the availability of essential supplies can create a culture of safety and infection prevention. In Liberia, the post-Ebola recovery plan emphasized, also, the integration of IPC into all health services, leading to a stronger health system [48].

Additionally, understanding the social pathways of infection spread and the conflicting human values in infection control is crucial for managing complex situations, such as the Ebola epidemic in Upper West Africa. Richards et al. [17], using case study data from central Sierra Leone, highlighted important social factors that must be considered in efforts to control the epidemic.

5.8 Conclusion

IPC in nonconventional settings requires a multifaceted approach that combines innovation, community engagement, and policy advocacy. By learning from past and present experiences, healthcare providers and policymakers can develop tailored strategies to mitigate the impact of infectious diseases and improve health outcomes in vulnerable populations worldwide in the future. Effective collaboration among healthcare providers, humanitarian organizations, and local authorities is essential for sustaining IPC efforts in these challenging environments.

References

1. World Bank. Fragility, conflict & violence [Internet]. The World Bank; 2024. Available from http://www.worldbank.org/en/topic/fragilityconflictviolence/overview. Last access 14/07/24
2. Leatherman S, et al. Quality health care in extreme adversity-an action framework. Int J Qual Health Care. 2019:mzz066. https://doi.org/10.1093/intqhc/mzz066.
3. World Health Organization. Quality of care in fragile, conflict-affected and vulnerable settings: taking action. World Health Organization; 2020. Available at: https://iris.who.int/handle/10665/337842
4. Allegranzi B, et al. Burden of endemic health-care-associated infection in developing countries: systematic review and meta-analysis. Lancet. 2011;377(9761):228–41. https://doi.org/10.1016/S0140-6736(10)61458-4.
5. World Health Organization (WHO). Major Trauma backpack 2021. Available at https://www.who.int/emergencies/emergency-health-kits/major-trauma-backpack. Last accessed 04/05/2024.
6. Muhrbeck M, et al. Predicting surgical resource consumption and in-hospital mortality in resource-scarce conflict settings: a retrospective study. BMC Emerg Med. 2021;21:94. https://doi.org/10.1186/s12873-021-00488-2.
7. World Health Organization. Regional Office for the Western Pacific. Considerations for community hand hygiene practices in low-resource situations. WHO Regional Office for the Western Pacific; 2020. Republished in May 2022 without changes. Available at https://iris.who.int/handle/10665/332382
8. Nguyen D, et al. Incidence and predictors of surgical-site infections in Vietnam. Infect Control Hosp Epidemiol. 2001;22(8):485–92. https://doi.org/10.1086/501938.

9. World Health Organization & United Nations Children's Fund (UNICEF). Infection prevention and control and water, sanitation and hygiene measures in health-care settings and shel-
   ters/congregate settings in Gaza: technical note, 22 February 2024. World Health Organization.
   Available at https://iris.who.int/handle/10665/376082
10. Dureab FA. The impact of conflict on the health situation in Yemen 2015. J Emerg Med Trauma
    Acute Care. 2016;31 https://doi.org/10.5339/jemtac.2016.icepq.31. International Conference
    in Emergency Medicine and Public Health – Qatar (PDF) The impact of conflict on the health
    situation in Yemen 2015. Available at: https://www.researchgate.net/publication/315718780_
    The_impact_of_conflict_on_the_health_situation_in_Yemen_2015#fullTextFileContent. Last
    accessed on July 2024
11. Checchi F, et al. Public health information in crisis-affected populations: a review of meth-
    ods and their use for advocacy and action. Lancet. 2017;390(10109):2297–313. https://doi.
    org/10.1016/S0140-6736(17)30702-X.
12. Sen K, et al. Syria: effects of conflict and sanctions on public health. J Public Health.
    2013;35(2):195–9. https://doi.org/10.1093/pubmed/fds090.
13. Médecins Sans Frontières. International activity report 2017. Available at: https://www.aerzte-
    ohne-grenzen.de/sites/default/files/msf-international-activity-report-2017.pdf
14. Islam MM, Yunus MY. Rohingya refugees at high risk of COVID-19 in Bangladesh. Lancet
    Glob Health. 2020;8(8):e993–4. https://doi.org/10.1016/S2214-109X(20)30282-5.
15. Ikram MS, et al. Communicable disease control in Afghanistan. Glob Public Health.
    2013;9(Suppl 1):S43–57. https://doi.org/10.1080/17441692.2013.826708.
16. Miller NP, et al. Community health workers during the Ebola outbreak in Guinea, Liberia,
    and Sierra Leone. J Glob Health. 2018;8(2):020601. https://doi.org/10.7189/jogh.08.020601.
    PMID: 30023054; PMCID: PMC6030670
17. Richards P, et al. Social pathways for Ebola virus disease in Rural Sierra Leone, and some
    implications for containment. PLoS Negl Trop Dis. 2015;9(4):e0003567. https://doi.
    org/10.1371/journal.pntd.0003567-.
18. McCarney S, et al. Using solar-powered refrigeration for vaccine storage where other sources
    of reliable electricity are inadequate or costly. Vaccine. 2013;31(51):6050–7. https://doi.
    org/10.1016/j.vaccine.2013.07.076.
19. Singhal G, et al. Mobile health clinics: mobilizing healthcare to reach the underserved. Glob
    Health Sci Pract. 2018;6(2):235–46.
20. Hollander JE, Carr BG. Virtually perfect? Telemedicine for COVID-19. N Engl J Med.
    2020;382(18):1679–81. https://doi.org/10.1056/NEJMp2003539. Epub 2020 Mar 11.-
21. World Health Organization. Global report on infection prevention and control. World Health
    Organization; 2022. Available at https://iris.who.int/handle/10665/354489
22. World Health Organization. Global strategy on infection prevention and control. World Health
    Organization; 2023. Available at https://iris.who.int/handle/10665/376751
23. Rizan C, et al. Environmental impact of personal protective equipment distributed for use by
    health and social care services in England in the first six months of the COVID-19 pandemic.
    J R Soc Med. 2021;114(5):250–63.
24. Chen Z, et al. A pandemic-induced environmental dilemma of disposable masks: solutions
    from the perspective of the life cycle. Environ Sci Process Impacts. 2022;24(5):649–74.
25. Sphere Association. The sphere handbook: Humanitarian charter and minimum standards in
    humanitarian response. 4th ed. Geneva; 2018. www.spherestandards.org/handbook
26. World Health Organization. Minimum standards and recommendations for medical teams
    responding to highly infectious disease outbreaks. World Health Organization; 2024. Available
    at https://iris.who.int/handle/10665/377995
27. Global Health Security Agenda. Global health security agenda [Internet]. Available from
    https://globalhealthsecurityagenda.org. Last access 21/07/24
28. Murphy RA, Chua AC. Prevention of common healthcare-associated infections in humani-
    tarian hospitals. In: Current opinion in infectious diseases, vol. 29. Lippincott Williams and
    Wilkins; 2016. p. 381–7.

29. Weintrob AC, et al. Active surveillance for asymptomatic colonization with multidrug-resistant gram-negative bacilli among injured service members—a three-year evaluation. MSMR. 2013;20(8):17–22.
30. Lowe H, et al. Challenges and opportunities for infection prevention and control in hospitals in conflict-affected settings: a qualitative study. Confl Health. 2021;15(1):94. https://doi.org/10.1186/s13031-021-00428-8. Erratum in: Confl Heal 2022 Jan 7;16(1):2. PMID: 34930364; PMCID: PMC8686079
31. George M, et al. 3D printed surgical instruments: the design and fabrication process. World J Surg. 2017;41(1):314–9. https://doi.org/10.1007/s00268-016-3814-5. PMID: 27822724; PMCID: PMC6287965
32. Sahloul MZ, et al. War is the enemy of health. Pulmonary, critical care, and sleep medicine in War-Torn Syria. Ann Am Thorac Soc. 2016;13(2):147–55. https://doi.org/10.1513/AnnalsATS.201510-661PS.
33. World Food Programme (WFP). Logistics cluster: annual report 2021. Available at https://logcluster.org/en/document/logistics-cluster-2021-annual-report; 2021
34. Matzopoulos R, et al. The impact of violence on health in low- to middle-income countries. Int J Inj Control Saf Promot. 2008;15(4):177–87. https://doi.org/10.1080/17457300802396487.
35. Yaacoub S, et al. Antibiotic resistance among bacteria isolated from war-wounded patients at the Weapon Traumatology Training Center of the International Committee of the Red Cross from 2016 to 2019: a secondary analysis of WHONET surveillance data. BMC Infect Dis. 2022;22:257. https://doi.org/10.1186/s12879-022-07253-1.
36. UNICEF. Yemen humanitarian situation report 2021. Available at https://www.unicef.org/media/117511/file/Yemen-Humanitarian-SitRep-End-of-Year-2021.pdf
37. Blyth DM, et al. Lessons of war: combat-related injury infections during the Vietnam War and Operation Iraqi and Enduring Freedom. J Trauma Acute Care Surg. 2015;79(4 Suppl 2):S227–35. https://doi.org/10.1097/TA.0000000000000768.
38. Tribble DR, et al. Infection-associated clinical outcomes in hospitalized medical evacuees after traumatic injury: trauma infectious disease outcome study. J Trauma. 2011;71(Suppl 1):S33–42. https://doi.org/10.1097/TA.0b013e318221162e.
39. Älgå A, et al. Infection with high proportion of multidrug-resistant bacteria in conflict-related injuries is associated with poor outcomes and excess resource consumption: a cohort study of Syrian patients treated in Jordan. BMC Infect Dis. 2018;18(233)
40. Harris E. Antimicrobial resistance is rising in Ukraine and neighboring areas. JAMA. 2024;331(2):101. https://doi.org/10.1001/jama.2023.25269.
41. World Health Organization. Global antimicrobial resistance and use surveillance system (GLASS). Retrieved July 28, 2024, from https://www.who.int/initiatives/glass
42. Almehdar H, et al. Antibiotic susceptibility patterns at the Médecins Sans Frontières (MSF) Acute Trauma Hospital in Aden, Yemen: a retrospective study from January 2018 to June 2021. JAC Antimicrob Resist. 2024;6(2):dlae024. https://doi.org/10.1093/jacamr/dlae024.
43. Ronat JB, et al. AMR in low-resource settings: Médecins Sans Frontières bridges surveillance gaps by developing a turnkey solution, the Mini-Lab. Clin Microbiol Infect. 2021;27(10):1414–21. https://doi.org/10.1016/j.cmi.2021.04.015.
44. Teicher CL, et al. Antimicrobial drug-resistant bacteria isolated from Syrian war-injured patients, August 2011–March 2013. Emerg Infect Dis. 2014;20:1949–51.
45. Murphy RA, et al. Multidrug-resistant chronic osteomyelitis complicating war injury in Iraqi civilians. J Trauma. 2011;71:252–4.
46. Chu K, et al. Rethinking surgical care in conflict. Lancet. 2010;375(9711):262–3. https://doi.org/10.1016/S0140-6736(10)60107-9.
47. Nnadi C, et al. Approaches to vaccination among populations in areas of conflict. J Infect Dis. 2017;216(Suppl 1):S368–72. https://doi.org/10.1093/infdis/jix175.
48. Bemah P, et al. Strengthening healthcare workforce capacity during and post Ebola outbreaks in Liberia: an innovative and effective approach to epidemic preparedness and response. Pan Afr Med J. 2019;33(Suppl 2):9. https://doi.org/10.11604/pamj.supp.2019.33.2.17619.jones.

Microbiology and Infectious Agents

6

Osman Sezer Cirit and Yeliz Tanrıverdi Çaycı

6.1 Introduction to Microbiology

Microscopic life originated billions of years ago from organic material found in the ocean waters and the gaseous cloud layers that surround the Earth. These microscopic organisms were the first living things on Earth and other forms of life evolved from them. Microbiology is the study of microscopic organisms and is a combination of the Greek words micros (small), bios (life), and logos (science). Despite the fact that microorganisms are such old and ancient creatures, the science of microbiology can be considered relatively young. Although humans have been on earth for billions of years, they only realized the existence of these microscopic creatures about 300 years ago. Since then, it has taken 200 years of dead time for microorganisms to be fully understood [1, 2].

Microorganisms of interest to medical microbiology can be divided into four groups. The first is eukaryotes, which means true nuclei. Eukaryotes are more evolved than the other group, prokaryotes, and include algae, protozoa, and fungi, which are relevant to microbiology. The second group of prokaryotes includes bacteria, and the third group includes viruses that do not have a classical cell structure and that do not replicate and have no metabolic activity unless they are in a living cell. In addition to these three groups, prions, which are responsible for some slowly progressive infectious diseases but, unlike their known living forms, do not contain nucleic acids, are among the structures of medical importance [1].

O. S. Cirit (✉)
Department of Microbiology, Gaziantep City Hospital, Gaziantep, Türkiye

Y. T. Çaycı
Department of Microbiology, School of Medicine, University of Ondokuz Mayıs, Samsun, Türkiye

6.2   Bacteriology

Bacteria originated millions of years ago and have not changed their seemingly simple structures for such a long time. However, what appears simple in shape and size is actually quite complex. Their size varies depending on the species, but averages around 1 µm. From the inside out, the bacterial cell contains the nucleus, cytoplasm, sometimes spores, cytoplasmic membrane, cell wall, sometimes capsule, pilus, and fimbriae. The bacterial nucleus consists of a single chromosome, circular, double-stranded DNA and can reach 1 mm in length. It has no nucleoplasm and no nucleus membrane. The chromosome is attached to the cell membrane through a region called the mesosome. The bacterial cytoplasm contains the nucleus, ribosomes, granules, plasmids. The cytoplasm is surrounded by a cytoplasmic membrane. Cytoplasmic membrane (inner membrane) is made up double-layered phospholipids and proteins. Bacteria, unlike eukaryotes, do not have sterols in their cytoplasmic membranes. The cytoplasmic membrane is making a selective permeability between the external environment and the bacteria exchange of substances or blocking it for some substances; the bacterium the provision of energy requirements, oxidative phosphorylation, i.e. respiration and cell is the synthesis of the wall. Just outside the cytoplasmic membrane is called the cell wall. The bacterial cell wall constitutes 10–40% of the dry weight of bacteria. All bacteria except Mycoplasmas have a cell wall. Cell wall synthesis takes place in the cytoplasmic membrane of bacteria. The peptidoglycan layer of the bacterial cell wall consists of linear peptidoglycan chains connected by side branches. This layer that is present in gram positive bacteria is much thicker than the gram-negatives and constitutes for about 50% of the dry weight of the bacteria [3]. The cell wall is not a homogeneous structure and contains different substances and layers. Because of these differences, bacteria are divided into two major groups, gram-negative and gram-positive, when stained with Gram stain. Crystal violet, lugol, alcohol, and safranin (or fuchsin) are used in Gram staining. Another function of the cell wall is to protect the bacterium against its internal pressure and to give it its shape. Bacteria are not all the same shape and have three main morphological structures. Round bacteria are called cocci (*Staphylococci, Streptococci*), rod bacteria are called bacilli (*Escherichia coli, Klebsiella pneumoniae*), and spiral or helical bacteria are called spiral (*Borrelia, Treponema, Leptospira*) [1, 3].

The outermost part of some bacteria has a sticky layer called the glycocalyx. If this layer of glycocalyx is thick, has a specific location within the bacterial structure, and is firmly attached to the cell wall, it is called a capsule. If this layer is thin, not tightly adherent to the cell wall, and easily detachable, it is called the slime layer. The most important role of the capsule in bacterial virulence is to prevent the activation of complement and consequently phagocytosis of the bacteria [3].

6.2.1   Pathogenesis

In order for an infection to occur, bacterial pathogens follow various strategies such as adhesion to host cells, tissue colonization, and in some cases intracellular proliferation after invasion into cells, and subsequent spread to other tissues or persist within the cell. Bacteria communicate between the host cell and the pathogen using monomeric adhesins/invasins or highly specialized macromolecular mechanisms, such as the Type III secretion system and the retractile Type IV pili. This communication between the host cell and the pathogen results in the destruction of host cell functions and the development of disease. Pathogenic bacteria cause diseases by two important mechanisms:

I. Invasion of cells: Invasion occurs through the colonization mechanism of microorganisms (adherence and proliferation), overcoming the host defense mechanism and production of extracellular substances.
II. Toxin production: Bacteria produce two types of toxins: exotoxins and endotoxins.

Bacteria colonize with its adhesion factors after colonization some bacteria invade and cause damage to the host cell with their toxins and enzymes. Bacterial toxins are the first virulence factors discovered in bacteria. Bacteria chemically produce two types of toxins: lipopolysaccharides in the cell wall of gram-negative bacteria (i.e., endotoxins) and proteins released by pathogenic bacteria (i.e., exotoxins) [1, 2].

Among gram-positive cocci, important human pathogens are *Staphylococcus aureus, Enterococcus faecium, Enterococcus faecalis,* and *Streptococcus pneumoniae*. Gram-negative bacteria include Enterobactarales and nonfermentative bacteria such as *Pseudomonas aeruginosa* and *Acinetobacter baumannii*, which are important nosocomial pathogens.

6.2.2   Emerging Bacteria

6.2.2.1   *Acinetobacter baumannii*

A. baumannii is a gram-negative nonfermentative bacterium. *Acinetobacter* species have been reported to be increasingly implicated in ventilator-associated pneumonia, especially in patients hospitalized in hospital intensive care units (ICU), and to increase the rate of the gram-negative infection agents in healthcare settings. *A. baumannii* is the most frequently isolated species from humans and the most frequently responsible for hospital infections. *Acinetobacter* strains, especially *A. baumanni* are resistant to multiple antimicrobial agents including carbapenems [4].

6.2.2.2 *Staphylococcus aureus*

Staphylococci are opportunistic pathogens for humans and animals. They colonize various parts of the human body. *S. aureus* colonizes the nasal mucosa of 70% of normal people, hospital workers and patients under treatment.

Staphylococcal infections: infections of the skin and mucous membranes, including abscesses, furuncles, cycosis (inflammation of the beard and hair follicles), carbuncles, panaris, hydroadenitis (inflammation of the sweat glands), bilepharitis (inflammation of the eyelids), inflammation of the tonsils, pharyngitis, peritonsillar abscess, and angina.

Methicillin-resistant staphylococcal infections are important because of their multi-resistance and nosocomial origin. Methicillin-resistant staphylococci: resistant to all betalactam antibiotics including nafcillin, oxacillin and cephalosporins, and vancomycin or teicoplanin should be used in treatment as they may also be resistant to aminoglycosides such as gentamicin, tobramycin, tetracycline, ciprofloxacin, and clindamycin [5, 6].

6.2.2.3 Enterobacteriaceae

Enterobacteriaceae is a heterogeneous family of bacteria found in the flora human and animal intestine and frequently isolated as pathogens from clinical specimens. Treatment of infections with Enterobacteriaceae members should be planned according to the antibiotic susceptibility of the bacteria.

Carbapenem resistance has recently gained importance in Enterobacteriaceae members due to infections with carbapenemase-producing Enterobacteriaceae. Although the epidemiologic characteristics of various carbapenem-resistant Enterobacteriaceae (CRE) species vary between regions, they are increasingly distributed worldwide. Although the treatment of infections due to these carbapenemase-forming bacteria is largely uncertain, mortality rates are high [7, 8].

6.2.2.4 *Pseudomonas aeruginosa*

P. aeruginosa is a major cause of hospital-acquired infections, especially in immune suppressed patients. Also in terms of general hygiene of the hospital, this bacterium is known to cause epidemics by contaminating water resources. *P. aeruginosa* quickly develops resistance due to its structural features and the effect of intense antibiotic stress in the hospital environment. The virulence factors determine the disease-causing capacity of the bacteria. These are factors such as structural components, toxins, and enzymes of *P. aeruginosa*. Both cellular and extracellular factors play a role in the virulence of *P. aeruginosa* [9].

6.2.2.5 Vancomycin-Resistant Enterococci (VRE)

The most prominent feature of enterococci today is their increasing resistance to antibiotics. The two most important species responsible for enterococcal infections are *E. faecalis* and *E. faecium*, with *E. faecalis* being more common. *E. faecium* is known to be more resistant to antimicrobials than *E. faecalis*. Because of this resistance, *E. faecium* constitutes most of the VRE isolates. Vancomycin is the last choice for the treatment of infections caused by resistance isolates. VRE was first identified in Europe in 1987 and became a worldwide pathogen in the following years. Today, it is one of the most feared pathogens in intensive care units. In meta-analyses conducted with VRE, a positive correlation between mortality and mortality was reported. Although there are differences between hospitals, vancomycin resistance rates of enterococci isolated from intensive care units are reported to be approximately 20% [10].

6.3   Mycology

6.3.1   Introduction to Mycology

Fungi are prevalent across the globe, with an estimated 1.5 million species inhabiting our planet; however, only a fraction is recognized as harmful to humans [11]. While they are crucial and beneficial players in ecosystems, aiding in the breakdown of organic materials as well as serving as a food source, fermentation agents, and sources of medicine, they also contribute to various infections affecting humans, animals, and plants [12].

The human body maintains a temperature of 37 °C, coupled with immune defenses and low redox potential within tissues, effectively warding off the majority of fungal invaders. The impact of fungal infections on public health and the economy is frequently underestimated, as shown by the absence of any focused initiatives on fungal diseases by the World Health Organization [11].

Each year, fungal infections result in approximately 1.5 million fatalities, with the population at risk of these infections on the rise [13]. The advent of multidrug-resistant pathogens and novel fungal species, alongside a deficiency in effective antifungal treatments, presents a considerable threat to public health [14].

6.3.2   The Structure of Fungi

Fungi are aerobic, eukaryotic, heterotrophic, spore-producing, nonmotile saprophytes that vary in form from tiny single-celled organisms referred to as yeasts to multicellular molds and intricate varieties that produce edible mushrooms.

Fungi, in line with their definition as widely prevalent organisms, are found in nearly every habitat, spanning from arid to humid areas, across tropical to temperate climates, from barren deserts to deep ocean depths, and existing as both symbionts and parasites.

Fungi can reproduce via both sexual and asexual methods. Those that reproduce solely through asexual means are classified as fungi imperfecti [11].

Distinctive features unique to fungi include a robust cell wall, primarily made up of chitin and glucans, which blocks many substances, such as antibacterial agents, along with the presence of ergosterol in their cellular membranes [11, 15].

Morphologically, the fungal kingdom is categorized into two main groups:

1. *Yeasts*: Under microscopic examination, they typically appear round or oval in shape, consisting of single-celled organisms that reproduce through budding, a process known as blastospore formation [13]. Certain species develop elongated and interconnected pseudohyphae that lack continuous attachments or do not demonstrate ongoing communication [11, 15]. Pseudohyphae can be identified from true hyphae by a constriction at the junction of two cells and the branching at that constricted area [13]. When viewed macroscopically, yeasts form moist and creamy colonies. The most notable yeasts of medical significance include *Candida* spp. and *Cryptococcus* spp. [11, 15].

2. *Molds*: Molds are filamentous and multicellular, showcasing complex structures that depend on their sexual or asexual reproductive processes [13]. The fundamental unit of a mold is the hypha, which is a filamentous structure that may be divided or undivided by septa [11, 15]. The hyphae, formed by the development and intertwining of branching hyphae, are referred to as mycelium [13]. Macroscopically, mycelium can be observed in both vegetative (basal) and aerial types. The portion of mycelium that remains on the surface of the medium in a colony on solid substrates is called aerial mycelium, which is connected to reproduction [11, 15]. Structures that form spores or conidia are present within aerial mycelium [13]. The arrangement and structure of conidia serve as valuable markers for the morphological identification of various molds [13, 15]. Fungi that reproduce sexually generate additional spore vessels, which are designated by different names, all aiding in the morphological classification of fungi. The mycelium extending into the medium is termed vegetative mycelium, which absorbs essential nutrients from the surrounding medium for sustenance [11, 15].

Dimorphic Fungi Beyond the two primary categories outlined above, certain fungi exist as yeasts within human tissues and specific environments at 37 °C, while they appear as molds at 26 °C (room temperature environment). *Histoplasma capsulatum*, *Blastomyces dermatitis*, *Coccidioides immitis* are important dimorfic fungi [11].

6.3.3 Epidemiology of Fungal Infections

The evolution of contemporary medicine closely mirrors the rise of invasive fungal infections. Historically, only a handful of fungi are recognized as pathogens in immunocompetent individuals, aside from dermatophytes and pathogenic dimorphic fungi. Superficial fungal infections account for the majority of all fungal infections. It is estimated that around 25% of the global population experiences fungal infections of the skin and nails during their lifetime. These conditions arise from dermatophytes and *Candida* species, commonly referred to as athlete's foot, ringworm, nail fungus, and similar maladies.

Acute or chronic superficial mucosal infections of the gastrointestinal and genital systems are also prevalent. It is estimated that approximately 50–75% of all women of reproductive age will encounter vulvovaginal candidiasis (VVC), and around 492 million women experience recurrent VVC (RVVC). With the advent of the Human Immunodeficiency Virus (HIV), incidences of oral and esophageal candidiasis have escalated significantly. While these diseases have personal and societal implications, they are generally manageable in the long term with suitable treatment. The issue of invasive fungal infections is gaining critical attention. The fungi most frequently associated with fatalities include *Candida*, *Aspergillus*, *Cryptococcus*, and *Mucorales*, with an average mortality rate of about 50%.

Several factors contribute to the heightened incidence of these infections in tropical regions: large populations that are economically disadvantaged and malnourished, restricted access to healthcare services, mismanagement of antibiotic prescriptions and steroid use, as well as the sale of these medications over the counter. Natural disasters, such as tsunamis, cyclones, and earthquakes, disrupt the soil significantly, leading to elevated spore levels in the environment and the establishment of saprophytic fungi due to injuries sustained during such calamities [11, 13].

The Factors That Predispose Individuals to Fungal Infections [13]

Prominent risk elements for various invasive fungal infections encompass:

- Neutropenia
- Cytotoxic chemotherapy
- Immunosuppressive therapy for autoimmune conditions
- Hematologic malignancies
- Cancer treatment
- HIV—AIDS
- Hematopoietic stem cell and solid organ transplants
- Young children or elderly individuals
- Diabetes
- Significant trauma and burns
- Prolonged antibiotic therapy
- Total parenteral nutrition
- Utilization of central vascular access devices

Medically significant mycoses can be categorized into four groups [13].

1. Cutaneous
2. Subcutaneous
3. Systemic
4. Opportunistic

6.3.4 Opportunistic Mycosis

In general, invasive fungal infections or opportunistic mycoses are believed to arise when the host's immunity is compromised. Both innate and adaptive immunity are crucial defenses against fungal pathogens. When cell-mediated immunity is impaired (as seen in HIV infections), diseases like cryptococcosis and certain endemic fungal infections proliferate. Conversely, invasive candidiasis, aspergillosis, and various mold infections are predominant during a decline in natural immunity or neutropenia (such as in cancer patients undergoing chemotherapy, organ transplant recipients). These infections can manifest as fungemia, invasive lung infections, central nervous system infections, disseminated infections, etc. [11].

6.3.4.1 Candidiasis
Species of *Candida* are microorganisms typically present as normal flora on human skin and mucosa, and their diseases are of endogenous origin. Through superficial invasions, they lead to candidiasis in the oral mucosa, genital regions, and skin, as well as onychomycosis due to nail involvement. The pathogen that most frequently causes fungal sepsis is *Candida* spp. *Candida* spp. accounts for 80% of all nosocomial fungal infections and 15% of all hospital-associated diseases [16, 17].

6.3.4.2 Cryptococcosis
C. neoformans is responsible for cryptococcosis, particularly cryptococcal meningitis, making it the most prevalent life-threatening fungal illness in AIDS patients. *C. neoformans* is an oval, budding yeast encased in a large polysaccharide capsule. This organism becomes pathogenic in humans following inhalation of spores from pigeon droppings, commonly found in soil. There is no transmission from person to person. Lung involvement may be asymptomatic or result in pneumonia [16, 17].

6.3.4.3 Aspergillosis
Among the species of *Aspergillus*, *Aspergillus fumigatus* is especially known for causing infections in the skin, eyes, ears, and lungs. It is identified by the formation of septate hyphae that branch in a V-shaped manner. This fungus is abundantly found in nature and infects humans via airborne conidia. It is the leading cause of fungal sinusitis and is particularly notorious for its ability to thrive in cavities created in the lungs due to tuberculosis. It forms "fungus balls" termed aspergillomas within these cavities. In culture, the spores of Aspergillus colonies display a distinctive structure by forming a radial chain [13, 16].

6.3.4.4 Mucormycosis
Mucormycosis is an illness caused by saprophytic molds (like Mucor and Rhizopus) that are prevalent in the environment. It invades tissues in immunocompromised individuals due to airborne transmission of asexual spores [16, 17].

6.3.5   Fungal Infection Immunity and Pathogenesis

Fungi are widely distributed throughout the environment, with some serving as resident or transient commensals within the human body. For coexistence, the human immune response must uphold a balance between fungal invasion and host defense.

When this equilibrium is disrupted, fungal infections may ensue. Both innate and adaptive immunity play vital roles in combating fungal infections [11].

6.3.6   Fungal Virulence

Several mechanisms contribute to fungal pathogenesis. Fungi produce various virulence factors that assist in adhesion, tissue invasion, and evasion of immune defenses. The rigid cell wall of fungi, made up of diverse polysaccharides, serves multiple purposes. It primarily protects the organism from external environmental stresses while also maintaining resistance against turgor pressure during hyphal growth. In numerous pigmented fungi, melanin helps in evading immune responses by blocking chitin, dectin 1, and subsequent cytokine synthesis. Additionally, the development of pseudohyphae and true hyphae within tissues facilitates tissue invasion [13].

6.4   Parasitology

6.4.1   Introduction to Parasitology

Human parasitic diseases are caused by entities classified as protozoa (unicellular entities), flatworms (including trematodes and cestodes), roundworms (also known as nematodes), along with various arthropods (such as insects, ticks, and mites). The prevalence of these parasitic diseases in tropical and subtropical regions is influenced by factors such as poor living conditions, insufficient financial resources for treatment and disease management, inadequate nutrition, a lack of health education, cultural and ethnic practices that may favor parasite transmission, environmental factors, and compromised immune systems [18].

6.4.2   Classification of Parasites

6.4.2.1 Protozoa
Protozoa are composed of a single cell, and they may have a defined shape or not. Certain groups possess specialized locomotion structures (including flagella, pseudopodia, and cilia). They obtain nutrients through phagocytosis, pinocytosis, and/or absorption. Some species can exist freely, while others exhibit parasitic behavior when conditions permit (e.g., Acanthamoeba, Naegleria) [19].

The phyla that harbor human parasites include the following:

Sarcomastigophora
These organisms feature free-living and parasitic representatives. They are categorized into two distinct categories: (1) Sarcodina (rhizopoda): They navigate using pseudopods and are made up of amoebas. (2) Mastigophora (flagellates): Their

means of locomotion is flagella, and the quantity of these flagella differs across various genera and species. Examples of these genera include *Trypanosoma* and *Leishmania* [19].

Apicomplexa
They lack specific structures for movement. Their main feature is the apical complex, which plays a role in entering host cells. These organisms are all parasites, including *Plasmodium* and *Toxoplasma gondii* [19].

Ciliophora (ciliates)
They move using cilia. There's only one genus that lives inside humans: *Balantidium coli* [19].

Microspora
These intracellular parasites can infect almost everyone but are more successful in those with weakened immune systems. They stand out from other protozoa by having spores between their life stages and are considered ancient eukaryotes [19].

6.4.2.2 Helminths (Worms)
Their bodies are composed of multiple cells and have complex organs. They are divided into three main groups based on their medical importance: flatworms (Trematodes and cestodes), roundworms (Nematodes), and tapeworms [19].

Trematodes
They have a single body and are flattened, leaf-like in shape. They lack a body cavity and no anus in their digestive system, with their mouth acting as both a food intake and an exit point. Except for the Schistosomatidae family, most species are hermaphrodites, with some being free-living [19].

Cestodes
Their bodies are divided into three sections: head (scolex), neck, and rings. They are flattened and resemble a long strip of rings. They lack a digestive system or body cavity and are hermaphrodites. All species are parasites, living inside humans and other organisms [19].

Nematodes
Their bodies are cylindrical and have false body cavities. They have a complete digestive system that runs from mouth to anus. Males and females are separate, and there are also free-living species [19].

6.4.2.3 Annelida
Within this category, only leeches play a significant role in human health. Their bodies are composed of a single segment. They possess a sucker at both the front and back, along with a true internal cavity. They have a fully developed digestive system and are capable of self-reproduction.

6.4.2.4 Acanthocephalans (Acanthocephala)
Their bodies are structured as a single, cylindrical segment. They feature a spiny proboscis at the front. They have a false internal cavity and their sexes are distinct [19].

6.4.2.5 Arthropods (Arthropoda)
The anatomy of arthropods, which are crucial for human health, can be one, two, or three segments. They have true internal cavities. Their outer covering is a hard exoskeleton of chitin, and they possess jointed limbs. Their digestive systems are fully developed, and they exhibit sexual dimorphism. Additionally, there are species that are free-living [19].

6.4.3 Epidemiology of Parasitic Infections

HAIs predominantly impact patients who have compromised immune systems, often due to factors such as age (infants, the elderly), surgical conditions, diabetes, the use of immunosuppressive medications, and AIDS. The primary source of these infections is often the patients themselves, serving as reservoirs for pathogens; however, other potential sources include healthcare staff and visitors, food, water, blood donations, organ transplants, and insects [20].

6.4.3.1 Blood Transfusion/Solid Organ Transplantation
Infections related to healthcare settings and those mediated by blood transfusions from pathogens like *Toxoplasma gondii*, *Plasmodium* spp., *Babesia* spp., *Trypanosoma cruzi*, *Leishmania* spp., and microfilariae are well documented.

The protozoan infection most frequently associated with blood and blood product transfusions is *Plasmodium falciparum*, with *P. vivax* following. While this issue is prevalent in endemic regions, transmission can also occur between hospitalized individuals where physical barriers, like bed nets, are absent.

In solid organ transplantation, *Toxoplasma gondii* infections are the most prevalent parasitic infections; transmission via tachyzoites can happen if the infection is present shortly before organ donation, whereas bradyzoites can be transmitted even if the donor was infected long before the transplantation.

These infections can result in fatal conditions such as encephalitis, myocarditis, pneumonitis, chorioretinitis, and generalized lymphadenopathy in immunocompromised individuals, particularly after heart and lung transplants, but they have also been noted post-kidney transplants [20, 21].

6.4.3.2 Person-to-Person Contact
Hand hygiene within hospitals has historically been a concern, and while adherence among healthcare providers has markedly improved, it continues to present some challenges. Enterobiasis ranks as the leading helminth infection, particularly among school-aged and preschool children, and humans are the exclusive hosts of *E. vermicularis*. The foremost route of infection is person-to-person transmission,

including autoinfection via contaminated hands, as well as through contaminated objects (e.g., toys) or via inhalation (e.g., during bed making).

The itch mite *Sarcoptes scabiei*, an extraintestinal parasite transmitted through direct contact between persons, is also significant. Scabies represents a widespread parasitic skin condition affecting over 130 million individuals globally at any given time. The mites burrow into the skin's surface, where their excrement incites a host immune reaction that results in severe itching [20].

Within hospital settings, patients with weakened immune systems or elderly residents in nursing homes who harbor unrecognized crusted (Norwegian) scabies are primary sources of *S. scabiei* transmission. Infestations of the itch mite *S. scabiei* significantly contribute to healthcare-associated infections, with the resulting scabies disease spreading directly via skin contact or through sexual interactions. Notably, Norwegian or crusted scabies is linked to impairments in cell-mediated immunity, such as those seen in HIV/AIDS [21].

6.4.3.3 Water/Food

The transmission of infections through contaminated water is the most prevalent method. Occasionally, person-to-person transmission occurs, while foodborne transmission is infrequent [21]. As a general guideline, drinking water within hospitals does not usually pose a threat to typical patients. However, for high-risk individuals (immunocompromised, patients in intensive care), hospital tap water may serve as a source of nosocomial infections, as can inadequate hygiene practices in hospital kitchens [20].

Enteric protozoa are the leading causes of healthcare-associated outbreaks; numerous parasite species can be transmitted to humans via drinking water or food, including *Entamoeba histolytica*, *Giardia* spp., *Cryptosporidium* spp., *Cyclospora cayetanensis*, *Cystoisospora belli*, *Balantidium coli*, *Toxoplasma gondii*, *Trypanosoma cruzi*, *Dibothriocephalus latum*, *Taenia* spp., *Fasciola hepatica*, *Clonorchis sinensis*, *Opisthorchis* spp., and *Trichinella* spp.. Additionally, free-living amoebae like *Naegleria fowleri* and *Acanthamoeba* spp. can infect humans upon contact with water. Reports of hospital infections linked to these water- or foodborne parasites exist [20, 21].

Helminths have the potential to trigger localized outbreaks among recipients of solid organ transplants. These infections are commonly linked to the contamination of food or water. Enteric helminth parasites that can spread from one individual to another include *Enterobius vermicularis*, *Strongyloides stercoralis*, and *Hymenolepis nana*. Additional roundworms, such as hookworm, trichuris, and toxocara species, also pose a risk for outbreaks if conditions allow for fecal contamination in healthcare settings (e.g., recreational sites) and enable the maturation of helminth eggs. Patients who excrete *Taenia solium* proglottids within a hospital context represent a significant potential source of infection. *S. stercoralis* can lead to hyperinfection in individuals undergoing prolonged immunosuppression, particularly those on steroid therapy and those infected with HIV or HTLV-1. *Cryptosporidium* spp. constitutes a significant contributor to diarrhea within the HIV-affected population. Free-living amoebae in hospital water systems and oxygen humidifier reservoirs have been shown to be an important reservoir of pathogens such as *Legionella pneumophilia* [21].

6.4.3.4 Arthropods

Possible infections linked to healthcare environments caused by ectoparasites encompass pediculosis, scabies, mites, and myiasis. The involvement of insect larvae and mites as pathogens in nosocomial infections predominantly pertains to ailments instigated by fly larvae (maggots) that thrive in necrotic tissue or at regions of secretion or excretion in anatomical cavities. Myiasis acquired in hospitals is frequently observed worldwide, where invading maggots present not only a medical concern on their own but can also exacerbate lesions caused by the maggots and transmit additional pathogens. Moreover, cockroaches possess the capacity to disseminate bacteria.

Given the substantial pigeon populations in numerous urban areas, the poultry red mite *Dermanyssus gallinae* poses a challenge in healthcare facilities. Hospital-related infestations have been linked to pigeon nests adjacent to hospital windows, for instance, or pigeons resting in or on air conditioning systems [20].

The pigeon mite, *Dermanyssus gallinae*, has been involved in outbreaks acquired within healthcare facilities. Typically, these mites originate from pigeon nesting areas situated near ventilation systems or outdoor cooling units [21].

Lice are obligate parasites found across the globe. The three commonly encountered varieties are *Pediculus humanus capitis* (head louse), *Pediculus humanus corporis* (body louse), and *Phtirus pubis* (pubic louse). The primary mode of transmission for head lice is through direct head contact, with other methods including the sharing of hats, combs, towels, and bedding. As body lice are established vectors for diseases such as *Borrelia recurrentis*, *Rickettsia prowazekii*, and *Bartonella quintana*, the admission of a patient infested with body lice into a hospital can facilitate the spread of both the lice and potential bacterial infections. While no cases of hospital-acquired infections related to pubic lice have been documented, inadequate hygiene can result in infestations within healthcare environments [20].

6.5   Viruses

Viruses do not have a cellular structure and are infectious agents, have a simpler structure compared to other organisms. A complete virus particle consists of a capsid, which has a protein structure and has a protective function, and nucleic acid sequences wrapped in it or in the capsid. A complete virus particle capable of infection is called a virion. For the first time in 1892, Dmitri Ivanowski (Russia) discovered an organism that retained its infectivity despite being filtered from plants. Martinus Beijerinck (Netherlands), a botanist, is another important researcher who contributed to the identification of viruses [22]. It took time to realize that viruses are the causative agents of many diseases since they are too small to be visible to the eye and to identify the agents. Smallpox vaccine was administered by Edward

Jenner (England) in 1796 and rabies vaccine was developed by Louis Pasteur (France) in 1885, but neither of them had seen the disease agent [23].

Replication of viruses was first made possible by the production of smallpox vaccinia virus (vaccinia) in cell culture in 1913. In 1928, chick embryos were used as another vehicle for the production of viruses. In 1940 and afterwards, poliovirus, the causative agent of poliomyelitis, could be easily produced in cell cultures and shown in electron microscopes with modern technology, and the science of virology developed rapidly and the causative virus of many diseases was identified. Unlike other organisms, viruses cannot produce copies of themselves. This causes them to be described as "cell parasites" rather than "living organisms." They have no organelles to synthesize their own energy or to synthesize proteins. Unlike known viruses, mimivirus and megavirus, which have been discovered in waters in recent years, are viruses that are large enough to be seen in light microscope and whose disease-causing effects have not yet been identified [24].

In the last hundred years, epidemics caused by many viruses have been on the world agenda, leading to the death or disability of many people. Influenza virus (influenza), poliovirus (polio), Ebola virus (haemorrhagic fever), HIV (AIDS), CCHF-V (Crimean-Congo haemorrhagic fever), norovirus (diarrhea), human papilloma virus (cervical cancer) have been on the world agenda.

Since they are effective by settling inside the cells, the success rate in the treatment of virus diseases may be low. Protection methods from these agents are cheap and the most effective ways to prevent their spread. The number of people sickened worldwide has decreased with successful vaccine applications. Smallpox was the first infectious agent to be eliminated in the world as a result of vaccination. Polio and measles vaccinations have dramatically reduced the number of patients. Hepatitis B, rubella, mumps, chickenpox, yellow fever, tick-borne encephalitis agent virus, rotavirus, human papillomavirus have achieved successful results with the use of vaccines worldwide [24].

6.5.1 Structure of the Viruses

A complete virus particle capable of infection is called a virion. The virion basically consists of a capsid and nucleic acid structure, which is defined as the nucleocapsid. The capsid consists of protein subunits called "capsomers" and protects the nucleic acid from environmental conditions. Capsid structures of viruses can form geometric structures. The helical structure like a coiled spring is called "helical symmetry," the equilateral triangular shape is called "icosahedral symmetry," and the mixed structures are called "complex symmetry." Capsomers are synthesized by the host cell according to the nucleic acid sequences carried by the virus.

Viruses carry a single type of nucleic acid. Viruses are defined as "haploid" when the nucleic acid, defined as DNA or RNA, is carried in a single copy, except in retroviruses. Some viruses can carry more than one different nucleic acid fragment defined as "segment." The best example of this is influenza viruses, which can form new mixtures of nucleic acid fragments between viruses at different periods, resulting in influenza strains that synthesize new antigens. This phenomenon creates pandemics (major epidemics) that affect the whole world. Nucleic acid can be in a ring structure or in a chain structure. Unlike other organisms, virus nucleic acids can be single- or double-stranded RNA or DNA. Parvoviruses carrying single-stranded DNA and rotaviruses carrying double-stranded RNA are good examples of these differences [24].

In addition, hepatitis B virus differs in that part of the double-stranded DNA part is missing the opposite chain and partly single-stranded [24]. RNA viruses can be defined as positive or negative polarity according to the characteristics of the nucleic acid in their structure. Since the nucleic acid structure of RNA viruses with positive polarity shows mRNA similarity, protein synthesis can be initiated after entering the host cell. In order for protein synthesis to start in negative polarity RNA viruses, mRNA synthesis must be performed with the polymerase enzyme in the virion. Poliovirus is a good example of positive polarity RNA viruses, and since its nucleic acids alone can initiate protein synthesis, molecular test samples separated from its capsid in laboratories are also considered infectious [25].

Some viruses are surrounded by an "envelope" outside the capsid structure. The envelope is derived from the membranes of the host cell into which the virus enters and has a lipid and protein structure. The envelope may also contain glycoproteins of the virus. These sugary proteins serve as attachment sites to the host cell, while those defined as hemagglutinins can cause erythrocytes to adhere to each other. There are also glycoproteins with different functions. The envelope does not provide additional resistance to viruses; on the contrary, since it is sensitive to detergents and low pH, solvents such as alcohol, ether, and acid media inactivate viruses with envelopes. The space between the envelope and the capsid is called "tegument" and in this space there are viruses carrying some enzymes related to replication. For example, RNA polymerase for replication of mRNAs in viruses containing negative polarity RNA genome and reverse transcriptase enzymes enabling synthesis of DNA copy from viral RNA in retroviruses can be given [26].

6.5.2 Virus Infections

Viruses initiate their infections by entering the body from areas where they have receptors they recognize. Respiratory tract, blood, gastrointestinal system, genito-urinary tract, and mucous membranes are important entry routes of viruses. Since some viruses are very sensitive to dryness and heat, it is very difficult to be infected by using common items. Since they can preserve their properties in body fluids, transmission is frequently carried out through body fluids. In addition, viral infections transmitted from the pregnant mother to the fetus in the early stages of pregnancy can cause significant structural defects in the fetus. Depending on the nature of the host immune system, viral infections can be terminated by the action of interferon. Cytotoxic T lymphocytes also play an important role in the elimination of virus-infected cells [27].

Antibodies produced by the body against viruses can react with viruses and form deposits in the blood vessels, leading to muscle spasm or dysfunction in organs such as the kidneys. Viruses can cause chronic infections and some can cause cancer in the host. Epstein-Barr virus is associated with nasopharyngeal cancer and Burkitt lymphoma, herpesvirus type 8 with Kaposi's sarcoma, hepatitis B and C viruses with liver cancer and human papilloma virus with cervical cancer [28].

6.5.3 Viroids

They are nucleic acid sequences without protein structures that can only be effective in plants. Viroids are naked single-stranded RNA structures of 300–400 nucleotides in length and can spread between plants. No animal disease has yet been identified by viroids [24].

6.5.4 Prions

"Prion" proteins, which have no nucleic acid structure but are recognized to be capable of altering the structure of cell proteins in the areas where they are localized, are the most important agents of Creutz-Feldt-Jakob disease in humans. They are particularly concentrated in brain tissue and, after a long period of inactivity, can cause changes in personality and behavior that can lead to death. Since they are resistant to detergents and high temperatures, care must be taken to prevent prion infection during sterilization steps in health care. Treatment with sodium hydroxide and sterilization at high pressure and 134 °C should be applied especially for materials that will come into contact with the brain [29].

6.5.5 Coronaviridae

The family Coronaviridae and the genus coronavirus are enveloped, helically symmetric, single-stranded RNA viruses. They are so named because of the corona-like appearance of the virions when viewed with an electron microscope.

Coronaviruses are the second most common cause of the common cold. In 2002, a new type of coronavirus was the causative agent of severe acute respiratory syndrome, also known as SARS, which spread to Hong Kong and the rest of the world. The virus that causes the disease, which is characterized by high fever, pneumonia and acute respiratory distress syndrome (ARDS) in some patients and has a mortality rate of around 10%, has been named SARS-related Coronavirus (SARS-CoV). In 2012, a new coronavirus was identified in a patient who died of severe respiratory failure and was named Middle East Respiratory Syndrome Coronavirus (MERS-CoV).

Cases of pneumonia of unknown cause in Wuhan, China, in December 2019 have been reported. A new coronavirus has been detected in respiratory tract samples of patients has been identified. This new coronavirus, SARS-CoV-2, and the condition caused by COVID-19 has been named SARS-CoV2.

The outbreak has spread rapidly around the world and the WHO declared the situation a pandemic on March 11, 2020.

COVID-19 presents with a wide clinical spectrum ranging from asymptomatic patients to septic shock and multiple organ failure. Mild cases have mild symptoms such as dry cough, fever, sore throat, headache, but not severe symptoms such as respiratory distress. Moderate cases have respiratory symptoms such as cough, shortness of breath and rapid breathing, but no signs and symptoms of severe disease progression. Severe disease includes severe pneumonia, ARDS, sepsis, and septic shock [30, 31].

6.5.6 Retroviridae

Retroviruses have very specific replication. They require the enzyme RNA-dependent DNA polymerase (reverse transcriptase) to synthesize DNA from RNA.

The most important virus in this family is undoubtedly HIV. In the late 1970s and early 1980s in the United States of America, opportunistic infections in men who have sex with men and intravenous drug users, which were normally mild, unexpectedly resulted in death. This picture is called "acquired immune deficiency syndrome-acquired immune deficiency syndrome" and became known by the acronym AIDS. It was later discovered that the causative virus was HIV-1 and its variant HIV-2 viruses. The virus is spread sexually, through transfusions of blood and expore to body fluids and by infecting children born to infected mothers. The main target of the virus is CD4+ T lymphocytes, an important part of our immune system. The acute illness, characterized by infectious mononucleosis-like symptoms that occur when the virus first enters the body, has a mild course and then resolves. Over the years, as a result of viral replication, the death of CD4+ T lymphocytes and their numbers drop below certain levels, HIV infection turns into the clinical picture called AIDS. Opportunistic infections are more severe and can lead to virus-induced cancers such as Kaposi's sarcoma. Although HIV-1 itself can cause encephalopathy and dementia, most deaths are due to opportunistic infections [30, 32, 33].

6.6 Conclusion

The microbial world on our planet is extensive and varied. This encompasses the usual bacterial flora that resides on the skin and mucous membranes of humans. It is now widely acknowledged that microbial cells outnumber human cells in the human body. The gastrointestinal tract alone contains over ten times the number of microbial cells compared to the total number of human cells in the entire body. Currently, our grasp of the interaction between microbes and humans is, at best, basic. In a similar vein, the connection between humans and environmental microbes or surfaces is generally poorly understood, with the exception of some pathogenic microbes. Within the realm of infectious diseases and infection control, our focus often narrows to specific ailments caused by singular organisms. Traditionally, microbes have been viewed as harmful entities, largely due to the emphasis placed on disease rather than the interplay between human and microbial cells. The defensive role of numerous bacterial species inhabiting our surroundings has been significantly undervalued. In fact, these bacteria should be recognized as "Nature's Bioshield." Their relationship with their natural environments is potent and mutually beneficial. Since these organisms are prevalent in healthy individuals, their transfer from person to person holds minimal significance. We now recognize that disruptions to this bioshield caused by physical trauma, along with alterations stemming from antibiotic selection, represent the most critical risk factors for the emergence of infectious diseases, including those induced by multidrug-resistant bacteria and their spread in both healthcare and community settings. Person-to-person transmission was established even before the germ theory of disease gained traction. Historically, the practices of cleaning and sanitizing were in place long before germ theory was formally articulated; the focus was fundamentally on cleanliness. It is a reality that those we instruct to adhere to infection control protocols often lack a comprehensive understanding of the broader microbial landscape, complicating adherence to these practices. We assert that it is crucial to communicate to healthcare providers across all levels the importance of the microbial flora surrounding us, the elements that expose them to the risk of acquiring and transmitting disease-causing pathogens to vulnerable patients, particularly those affected by various factors such as age, immune deficiency, and comorbid conditions [34].

References

1. Procop GW, Church DL, Hall GS, Janda WM. Medical bacteriology: Taxonomy, morphology, physiology, and virulence. In: Koneman's color Atlas and textbook of diagnostic microbiology. 7th ed. Jones & Barlett. p. 173–82.
2. Tille PM. Bailey & Scott's diagnostic microbiology. In: Bacteriology, principles of identification. 15th ed. Elsevier, Can Underwrit; 2022. p. 208–20.
3. Murray PR, Rosenthal KS, Pfaller MA, editörler. Basustaoglu AC, geviri editörü. Tıbbi Mikrobiyoloji. Ankara: Atlas Kitapcılık; 2014. p. 553–661.
4. Aşık G. Acinetobacter baumannii Virülansının Açıklanmasında Güncel Yaklaşımlar. Mikrobiyol Bul. 2011;45(2):371–80.
5. Sancak B. MRSA Direnç Mekanizmaları: Dünyada Ve Türkiye'de Epidemiyolojisi. ANKEM Derg. 2012;26(Ek 2):38–47.
6. Levinson W. Tıbbi mikrobiyoloji ve immünoloji. Şener B, Esen B. (Çev.Editörleri). Güneş Kitabevi; 2018.
7. Tanrıverdi Çaycı Y, Bıyık İ, Çınar C, Birinci A. Karbapenem dirençli Enterobacteriaceae izolatlarının 2015-2018 yılları arasındaki antibiyotik direnci. Turk Mikrobiyol Cemiy Derg. 2020;50(3):134–40.
8. Morrill HJ, Pogue JM, Kaye KS, LaPlante KL. Treatment options for carbapenem-resistant Enterobacteriaceae infections. Open Forum. Infect Dis Ther. 2015;2:ofv050.
9. Bıyık İ, Çaycı YT, Atıgan EB, Birinci A. Identification of virulence resistance genes in *Pseudomonas aeruginosa* strains isolated from blood samples. J Biotechnol Strategic Health Res. 2022;6(1):64–9.

10. Parlak M, Binici İ, Çıkman A, Karahocagil MK, Bayram Y, Berktaş M. Vankomisine diren-
    çli enterokoklarda linezolid, tigesiklin ve daptomisin duyarlılığının E-Test yöntemiyle
    araştırılması. Dicle Med J. 2014;41(3):534–7.
11. Chakrabarti A, Sethuraman N. Introduction to medical mycology. In: Mora-Montes H, Lopes-
    Bezerra L, editors. Current progress in medical mycology. Cham: Springer; 2017. https://doi.
    org/10.1007/978-3-319-64113-3_1.
12. Chuku A. Effective diagnostic techniques in the identification of medically important fungi: a
    developing world perspective. ARRB. 2018;28(4):1–9. Article no.ARRB.43123
13. Cirit OS. Mikolojiye Giriş, Mantarların Yapısı ve Sınıflandırılması. In: Gazel D, editor. Sağlık
    Bilimlerinde Klinik Mikrobiyoloji. Ankara: Akademisyen Kitabevi; 2020. p. 219–32.
14. Arastehfar A, Wickeos BL, Ilkit M, Pincus DH, Daneshnia F, Pan W, Fang W, Boekhout
    T. Identification of mycoses in developing countries. J Fungi. 2019;5:90. https://doi.
    org/10.3390/jof5040090.
15. Winn W, Allen S, Janda W, Koneman E, Procop G, Schreckenberger P, Woods G. Koneman's
    color Atlas and textbook of diagnostic microbiology. 6th ed. New York: Lippincott Williams
    and Wilkins; 2006.
16. Levinson W. Review of medical microbiology and immunology. 11th ed. New York: McGraw-
    Hill; 2010.
17. Mantarların İR. Yapıları, Üreme Özellikleri ve Sınıflanması. In: Tümbay E, Ustaçelebi Ş, edi-
    tors. Temel ve Klinik Mikrobiyoloji. Güneş Kitabevi; 1999.
18. Bogitsh BJ, Carter CE, Oeltman TE. Symbiosis and parasitism. In: Human parasitology. 4th
    ed; 2013. p. 9. https://doi.org/10.1016/B978-0-12-415915-0.00001-7.
19. Miman Ö, Saygı G. Temel tıbbi parazitoloji. İstanbul tıp kitabevleri; 2008.
20. Fürnkranz U, Walochnik J. Nosocomial infections: do not forget the parasites! Pathogens.
    2021;10(2):238. https://doi.org/10.3390/pathogens10020238.
21. https://isid.org/wp-content/uploads/2019/07/ISID_GUIDE_PARASITES.pdf.   Chapter   last
    updated: February 2018
22. Sankaran N. On the historical significance of Beijerinck and his contagium vivum flu-
    idum for modern virology. Hist Philos Life Sci. 2018;40(3):41. https://doi.org/10.1007/
    s40656-018-0206-1.
23. Wagner KE, Hewlett JM. Basic virology. Blackwell Publishing; 2004. p. 1–10.
24. Engelkirk PG, Duben-Engelkirk J. Burton's microbiology for the health sciences. Philadelphia:
    Wolters Kluwer Health/Lippincott Williams & Wilkins; 2015. p. 45–57.
25. Wagner KE, Hewlett JM. Basic virology. Blackwell Publishing; 2004. p. 60–76.
26. Levinson W. Review of medical microbiology and immunology. McGraw-Hill; 2016.
    p. 226–31.
27. Altindis M, editér. Hemsireler icin mikrobiyoloji. Istanbul: Nobel Tip Kitabevleri; 2010.
    p. 253–63.
28. Levinson W. Review of medical microbiology and immunology. McGraw-Hill; 2016.
    p. 253–65.
29. Murray PR, Rosenthal KS, Pfaller MA, editors. Medical microbiology. 7th ed. Pennsylvania:
    Elsevier; 2012.
30. Payne S. Viruses. 1st ed. Elsevier; 2017.
31. Ryu WS. Molecular virology of human pathogenic viruses. 1st ed. Elsevier; 2016.
32. Robinson BJ, Pierson SLL, Virology C, Mahon CR, Lehman DC, Manuselis G, editörler.
    Textbook of diagnostic microbiology. Elsevier; 2011. p. 703–41.
33. Murray PR, Rosenthal KS, Pfaller MA, Basustaoglu AC, geviri editörü. Viroloji. In: Tıbbi
    Mikrobiyoloji. Ankara: Atlas Kitapçılık; 2014. p. 553–661.
34. El Lakkis I, Khardori N. The mighty world of microbes: an overview. Hospital Infect Prevent.
    2013:3–29. https://doi.org/10.1007/978-81-322-1608-7_1. PMCID: PMC7120817

Modes of Transmission

7

Noel Abela

7.1 Introduction

The modes of transmission of infectious diseases are a crucial aspect of infection prevention and control (IPC) strategies in healthcare settings. Understanding how pathogens spread from one host to another allows healthcare professionals to implement effective measures to break the chain of infection, thereby reducing the risk of healthcare-associated infections (HAIs). Transmission-based precautions, such as contact, droplet, and airborne precautions, are essential in addition to standard precautions to control the spread of highly transmissible or epidemiologically significant infections. These methods have become increasingly important, particularly during global health crises like the COVID-19 pandemic, where the understanding of respiratory transmission has evolved. By incorporating both standard and transmission-based precautions, healthcare environments can create safer spaces for both patients and healthcare workers, reducing the incidence of severe infections like MRSA, tuberculosis, and SARS-CoV-2.

7.2 Infection

7.2.1 What Is an Infection?

An infection is the invasion and multiplication of harmful microorganisms—such as bacteria, viruses, fungi, or parasites—within the body, which can result in disease. The human body is usually equipped with defences, such as the immune system, to combat these microbes. However, when these microorganisms evade immune

N. Abela (✉)
Faculty of Health Sciences, University of Malta, Msida, Malta
e-mail: noel.abela@um.edu.mt

© The Author(s), under exclusive license to Springer Nature Switzerland AG 2025   77
B. Oomen, S. Gastaldi (eds.), *Principles of Nursing Infection Prevention Control*,
Principles of Specialty Nursing, https://doi.org/10.1007/978-3-031-84469-0_7

responses, they can cause infections that may range from mild to life-threatening, such as sepsis (when the microorganisms invade the bloodstream, which can lead to multiorgan failure).

There are several types of infections depending on the pathogen involved:

- Bacterial infections are caused by bacteria, which are single-celled microorganisms that can live in various environments. Examples include Strep throat (caused by Streptococcus bacteria) and tuberculosis (caused by *Mycobacterium tuberculosis*).
- Viral infections occur when viruses enter the body, take over host cells, and reproduce. Common viral infections include influenza and SARS-CoV-2.
- Fungal infections are caused by fungi and can range from superficial infections, such as athlete's foot, to more severe infections in people with a weakened immune system.
- Parasitic infections are caused by parasites such as protozoa, helminths (worms), or ectoparasites (like lice). An example is malaria, which is caused by Plasmodium parasites.

7.2.2   Mechanism of Infection

Infections occur when pathogens overcome the body's defences and begin to multiply. The stages of infection typically involve the following:

1. *Colonization*: The pathogen adheres to host tissues and starts to multiply.
2. *Invasion*: The pathogen can enter deeper tissues or circulate in the blood.
3. *Evasion of host defences*: The pathogen uses various mechanisms to avoid immune detection.
4. *Tissue damage*: Infection may cause tissue damage either directly through microbial activity or indirectly by triggering an excessive immune response.

7.2.3   Types of Infections

- *Localized infection*: The infection remains confined to a specific part of the body, such as in a cut or wound.
- *Systemic infection*: The infection spreads throughout the body, often through the bloodstream, affecting multiple organs in a process known as sepsis.
- *Opportunistic infection* occurs when a normally harmless microbe takes advantage of a weakened immune system, such as in HIV/AIDS patients [1–3].

7.2.4   The Chain of Infection

If one had to ask what the common factor between fire and infections is, the answer would be that both SPREAD. A fire requires three elements (see Fig. 7.1). If one removes any element, the fire will be extinguished.

The chain of infection (Fig. 7.2) is like a fire; if we succeed in breaking the chain at any stage, then transmission will not occur.

Fig. 7.1 The three elements of fire. (Designed by author)

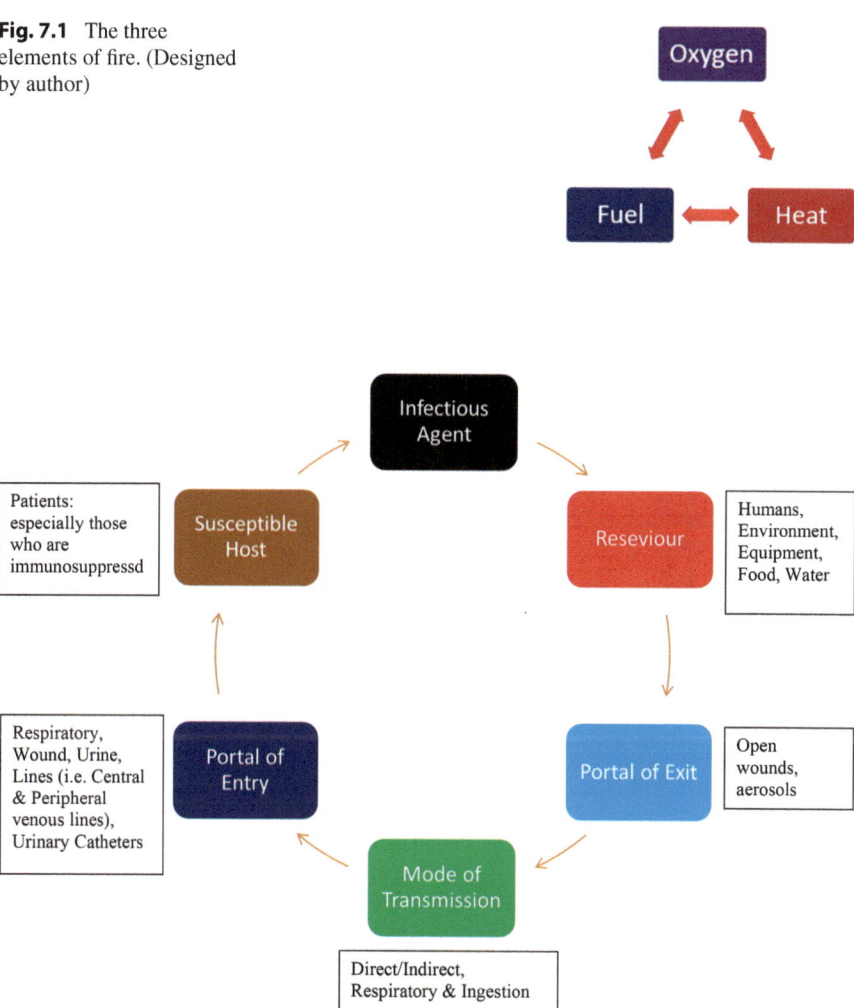

Fig. 7.2 The chain of infection. (Designed by Author)

7.3   The Infectious Agent

7.3.1   What Is the Infectious Agent?

The infectious agent can be bacteria, viruses, parasites, or fungi. These infectious agents are referred to as pathogens that are able to cause infections in the human body.

7.3.2   The Reservoir

A reservoir can be the environment, the hospital setting, water, people or animals like a rodent.

7.3.3   Portal of Exit

7.3.3.1 How Do the Infectious Agents Leave The Reservoir?
The infectious agents can leave the reservoir through open wounds, aerosols generated during sneezing or coughing and body fluids. For example, Influenza can be transmitted through coughing and sneezing.

7.3.4   Transmission

Transmission of the infectious agents can occur by direct or indirect contact e.g through unwashed hands, through inanimate objects and vectors.

7.3.5   Portal of Entry: How Does the Infectious Agent Enter the Body?

It can enter through inhalation, a break in the skin or mucus membranes, an insect bite, contaminated food or water.

7.3.6   Susceptible Populations: Who is Most Susceptible to These Infectious Agents?

Common susceptible populations are the very young, the very old and the immuno-suppressed. Occupational exposure should also be considered. The nonimmune group includes everyone who has not been previously exposed, nor has generated a specific immune response to the pathogen.

7.3.7   Standard Precautions

- Designed to reduce the risk of transmission of infection to the healthcare worker and from patient to patient [4].
- To be used with EACH and EVERY patient irrespective of whether their infectivity status is known or not [4].
- A risk assessment should determine what kind of PPE is needed.

The standard precautions consist of the following:

- Hand hygiene.
- Personal Protective Equipment (Mask, Gown, Apron, Visor/Goggles, Gloves).
- Proper disposal of sharps.
- Environmental Cleaning.
- Aseptic technique.
- Sterile instruments.
- Cough etiquette.

When standard precautions are not sufficient to stop the transmission of infections, transmission-based precautions need to be applied.

7.3.8   Transmission-Based Precautions

Transmission-based precautions are used in addition to standard precautions when a patient is confirmed to be infective to others and needs to be isolated in a single room or housed with other patients suffering from the same infection [4, 5].

Transmission-based precautions differ according to whether it is contact, droplet, or airborne transmission.

The World Health Organization has a free course, which is available at https://openwho.org/courses/IPC-TBP-EN

7.3.9   Examples of Microorganisms That Are Transmitted Through Contact, Droplets, and Airborne Environments

- Contact transmission.
- methicillin-resistant *Staphylococcus aureus* (MRSA), carbapenem-resistant Enterobacterales (CRE), extended-spectrum beta-lactamases (ESBLs)*, *Clostridioides difficile,*
- Droplet transmission: influenza, SARS-CoV-2 virus, common cold, meningitis.
- Airborne transmission—Tuberculosis**, Measles, Varicella.

*These organisms, such as *Escherichia coli* (*E. coli*) and *Klebsiella pneumoniae* (*K. pneumoniae*), are capable of producing enzymes called extended-spectrum beta-lactamases; these enzymes block certain antibiotics, such as penicillin and cephalosporins [6].

**This generally refers to pulmonary TB, as there are other forms of TB that are referred to as extrapulmonary TB. Extrapulmonary TB patients are often not contagious unless they have the following:

(a) In addition to extrapulmonary illness, pulmonary disease;
(b) extrapulmonary illness confined to the larynx or mouth cavity;
(c) Extrapulmonary illness characterized by an open lesion or abscess with a high organism concentration, particularly if the lesion or abscess has extensive drainage or if the drainage fluid is aerosolized.

Both pulmonary and extrapulmonary tuberculosis are common in people living with HIV [7].

7.4   Definition of Contact, Droplet, and Airborne Transmission

7.4.1   Definition of Contact Transmission

The physical transfer of infectious agents from an infected or colonized person to another susceptible person through contact or contact with blood or body substances without the need for an intermediary contaminated object or person is known as direct contact transmission [8].

7.4.2   Definition of Indirect Contact Transmission

The definition of indirect contact transmission is the spread of an infectious agent through a contaminated intermediate object to a susceptible host [8] (Table 7.1).

7.4.3   Definition of Droplet Transmission (Table 7.2)

Table 7.1 Definitions of contact transmission by different countries, the CDC and the WHO

World Health Organization (WHO) [4]	An infectious agent can spread by physical touch between a vulnerable host and other persons or objects. This process is known as contact transmission.
Centers for Disease Control and Prevention (CDC) [9]	By preventing direct or indirect contact with the patient or the patient's surroundings, contact precautions aim to stop the spread of infectious pathogens, particularly epidemiologically significant bacteria.
England [10]	The transfer of infectious pathogens by touch between individuals. Transmission that happens directly through skin-to-skin contact is referred to as direct contact transmission. Indirect contact transmission refers to the spread that takes place through touch with a contaminated object.
Australia [11]	When infectious agents are spread directly from one person to another without the use of a contaminated intermediary object or person, this is known as direct transmission. For instance, an infectious person's blood or other bodily fluids could come into touch with another person's mucous membrane or skin breaches. The introduction of an infectious agent through a contaminated intermediate object (fomite) or person is known as indirect transmission.

Designed by author

Table 7.2 Definitions of droplet transmission by different countries, the CDC, and the WHO

Canada, New Zealand, and Australia [8]	The concept of an expanded definition for droplet transmission is reflected in the guidelines from Canada, New Zealand, and Australia. These guidelines state that while droplet transmission can happen when droplets are expelled directly onto the mucosa of a susceptible person, it can also happen when infectious agents are transferred to mucosal surfaces through respiratory droplet-contaminated hands and surfaces.
England [10]	The transfer of infectious pathogens through droplets from one person to another.
Honk Kong [12]	Microorganisms that spread through respiratory droplets (diameter more than 5 μm), produced by coughing, sneezing, or talking patients
Ireland [13]	Direct contact with infected respiratory droplets on nearby people's mucosa or contact with contaminated surfaces that subsequently transfer infectious material to mucous membranes can both result in transmission to other people.
World Health Organization (WHO) [14]	Respiratory pathogens that are transmitted through large droplets
Centers for Disease Control and Prevention (CDC) [15]	Although some infectious agents spread through droplet transmission can also spread through direct and indirect contact pathways, droplet transmission is technically a type of contact transmission. Nevertheless, respiratory droplets containing infectious pathogens spread infection differently from contact transmission because they move straight from the infectious person's respiratory tract to the recipient's susceptible mucosal surfaces, usually over short distances, requiring face protection.

Designed by author

7.4.4 Definition of Airborne Transmission

According to international infection control guidelines, airborne transmission occurs when an infecting host's respiratory processes produce infectious "small" aerosol particles, also known as "droplet nuclei," which are inhaled [8].

A recent publication by the WHO explains the definition of airborne transmission. Further information can be found in Sect. 7.5.

7.4.4.1 Contact, Droplet, and Airborne Transmission: Examples of Organisms According to the Chain of Infection (Tables 7.3, 7.4 and 7.5)

Table 7.3 Contact transmission: examples of organisms according to the chain of infection

	Contact transmission chain of infection
Organism	Methicillin-resistant *Staphylococcus aureus* (MRSA) Carbapenemase producing organisms (CPOs)[a] Extended Spectrum Beta-Lactamases (ESBL's) like *Escherichia coli* (*E. coli*) and *Klebsiella pneumoniae* (*K. pneumoniae*) Vancomycin-resistant enterococci *Clostridioides difficile* (*C. difficile*)
Reservoir	Healthcare worker hands, patient care equipment, computers, inadequately cleaned and/or sterilized medical instruments and environmental surfaces, for example, furniture, bedrails.
Portal of exit	Indirect/direct contact
Transmission example	HCW does not perform HH after patient contact hence HCW gets MRSA on hands
Portal of entry	HCW empties the urinary bag and contaminates the urinary catheter system and MRSA/CRE will eventually ascends to the bladder
Susceptible host	Patient

Designed by the author
[a]Important for isolating patients with different enzymes separately, e.g., KPC, OXA, VIM, and NDM

Table 7.4 Droplet transmission chain of infection: examples of organisms according to the chain of infection

	Droplet transmission chain of infection
Organism	Influenza A/B, SARS-CoV-2 virus[a], common cold, mumps, meningococcal meningitis
Reservoir	Respiratory tract
Portal of exit	Nose and mouth
Transmission	Air, inanimate objects, and contaminated hands
Portal of entry	Mouth and respiratory tract
Susceptible host	Patient and healthcare workers

Designed by author
[a]During the COVID-19 pandemic, physical distancing was increased from 1 m to 2 m as an extra precautionary measure. In the new national infection prevention manual, from the United Kingdom, this number has decreased back to 1 m [16]

Table 7.5 Airborne transmission chain of infection: examples of organisms according to the chain of infection

	Airborne transmission chain of infection
Organism	Tuberculosis, measles, chickenpox[a]
Reservoir	Respiratory tract
Portal of exit	Nose and mouth
Transmission	Air, inanimate objects, and contaminated hands
Portal of entry	Mouth and respiratory tract
Susceptible host	Patient and healthcare workers

Designed by author

7.5   Through the Air

The World Health Organization published a report in 2024, "Global Technical consultation report on proposed terminology for pathogens that transmit through the air" [4].

The main goal of this worldwide technical consultation study is to reach a consensus on the nomenclature for infections that are potentially infectious to humans and are spread through the air. Experts from a variety of disciplines contributed their perspectives to this discussion. During the COVID-19 pandemic, there was a lack of consensus on the terms "airborne," "airborne transmission," "droplets" and "aerosols." This led to confusion as to which way the pathogen is transmitted; hence, there was a need for such a document to be published explaining these different terms in more detail.

"Through the air" can be conveyed as two descriptors (Figs. 7.3 and 7.4):

This WHO publication aims to change the accepted understanding of the term "infectious respiratory particles" (IRPs) by removing the rigid distinction between particle sizes and acknowledging the possibility of both short- and long-range transmission of smaller IRPs. In addition, the term "transmission through the air" serves as an umbrella term for the dissemination of IRPs via direct deposition as well as airborne means. The idea behind this is to streamline the mode of transmission, but more specialized socialization and training will be required for both the public and healthcare professionals.

This document should be viewed as a jumping-off point for more thorough conversations and evidence reviews, which will help implement the recommendations made here with a clearer definition of what is meant by "through the air."

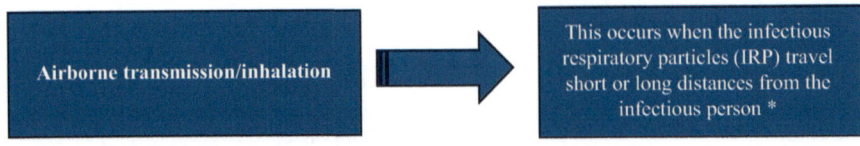

Fig. 7.3 (Designed by author)
*When the IRP travels, it depends on various factors, such as particle size, mode of expulsion, and environmental conditions

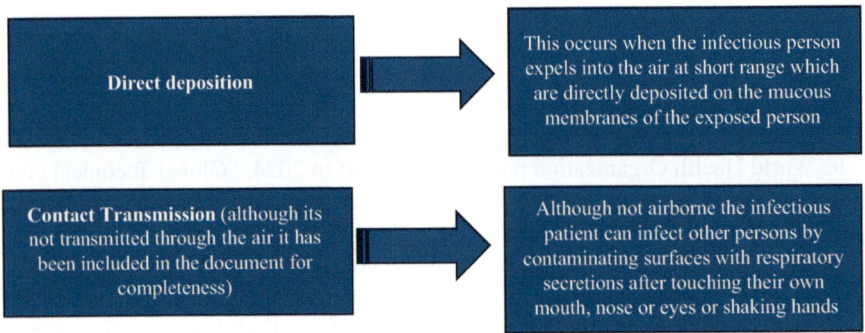

Fig. 7.4 (Designed by author)

7.6   Aerosol Generating Procedures

7.6.1   What Is the Definition of an Aerosol Generating Procedure?

Any medical and patient care technique that produces airborne particles (aerosols) is referred to as an aerosol-generating procedure (AGP). AGPs have the ability to create droplets smaller than 5 microns, which can travel a considerable distance and potentially infect someone if inhaled. As a result, AGPs increase the possibility that infections that typically spread through droplet transmission become airborne. The majority of AGPs are brief, sporadic, one-time occurrences. As a result, they would only present a risk of producing aerosols during those particular episodes. Any necessary safety measures would only be implemented while the AGP is being carried out. AGPs should be performed only in dire circumstances. Only the medical professionals required to perform the procedure should be present at the time that an AGP is being performed [18, 19].

7.6.2   Aerosol Generating Procedures (AGPs)

There is now more trustworthy literature that indicates which methods are indeed AGPs as a result of the increased research into AGPs during the COVID-19 epidemic. This has led to the removal of some procedures that were listed as AGPs in the past [20].

The most recent list of medical procedures by the UK document [20] thought to produce aerosols and increase the possibility of airborne transmission is as follows:

- awake* bronchoscopy (including awake tracheal intubation),
- Awake* ear, nose, and throat (ENT) airway procedures that involve respiratory suctioning.
- awake* upper gastrointestinal endoscopy,
- dental procedures (the use of high-speed or high-frequency devices for example ultrasonic scalers/high-speed drills),
- Induction of sputum.
- Respiratory tract suctioning**.
- Surgery or postmortem procedures (such as high-speed cutting/drilling) likely produce aerosols from the respiratory tract (upper or lower) or sinuses.
- Tracheostomy procedures (insertion or removal).

*Awake including conscious sedation (excluding anaesthetized patients with secured airway).

** The available evidence relating to respiratory tract suctioning is associated with ventilation. In line with a precautionary approach, open suctioning of the respiratory tract, regardless of its association with ventilation, has been incorporated into the current AGP list. Only open suctioning beyond the oropharynx is currently considered an AGP. Oral/pharyngeal suctioning is not considered an AGP [20].

7.6.3   Aerosol Generating Procedures That Have Been Removed from the AGP List

The following procedures are *NO LONGER considered to be AGPs*:

- Manual facemask ventilation.
- Endotracheal intubation and extubation (in anesthetized patients).
- Noninvasive ventilation (NIV)—including CPAP and BIPAP.
- High-flow nasal oxygenation (HFNO).
- Flexible bronchoscopy in an anesthetized/paralyzed patient.
- Supraglottic airway insertion, use, and removal.

7.6.4   Aerosol Generating Procedures and COVID-19

A recent document published by the WHO on 9th October 2023 suggests "using airborne precautions while performing aerosol-generating procedures (AGPs) and, on the basis of a risk assessment*, when caring for patients with suspected or confirmed COVID-19" [21].

* The risk assessment should consider the following factors: the activity (procedure), the setting (patient care environment), and the patient [21].

Performing AGPs on COVID-19 patients without FFP2(N95)/FFP3 carries a higher risk for frontline healthcare workers in becoming infected with COVID-19 [22].

7.6.5 Airborne Precautions During Aerosol Generating Procedures Including COVID-19

The certainty of the evidence was assessed as extremely low since there is no direct information about the effectiveness of respirators versus medical masks in preventing SARS-CoV-2 infection when performing AGPs or in environments where AGPs are often conducted (Table 7.6).

7.6.6 Respirators N95/N99 and Fit Check

Single use N95/FFP2 (Fig. 7.6) respirators are the most used worldwide; however, some European institutions recommend the use of N99/FFP3 respirators during aerosol generating procedures. The UK Health and Safety Executive guiding principle is to reduce the risk to "as low as reasonably possible."

The use of respirators especially when performing aerosol generating procedures is of paramount importance as they offer protection against infections transmitted through the airborne route. However, every time that a healthcare worker wears a respirator, a fit check should be done to ensure that there are no air leakages making sure that the wearer has a good facial seal [23]. That's why a surgical mask (Fig. 7.5) is not sufficient when performing aerosol generating procedures as they do not offer complete fit without air leakages (Fig. 7.5).

During the COVID-19 pandemic, healthcare workers became infected during the care of infected patients with SARS-CoV-2 while performing aerosol generating procedures. The reason for this is due to multiple factors such as low supply of N95/

Table 7.6 Airborne precautions during AGPs

Airborne precautions during AGPs	1. Put the patient in an AIIR[a], preferably with 12 air changes per hour.
	2. Put on a respirator (such as the N95, FFP2, or FFP3) before going inside the patient's room, and take it off when you're done.[b]
	3. Verify the seal on your respirator and wash your hands both before and after using one.
	4. Make use of specialized or disposable patient care equipment
	5. If transit is required, advise the patient to wear a medical mask, practice good respiratory hygiene, and cough politely.

Adapted from infection prevention and control in the context of COVID-19: a guideline, 21 December 2023 [Internet]. www.who.int. Available from: https://www.who.int/publications/i/item/WHO-2019-nCoV-IPC-guideline-2023.4
[a]Airborne infection isolation room
[b]Strong recommendation for, very low certainty evidence

Fig. 7.5 Surgical mask. (Photo taken by author)

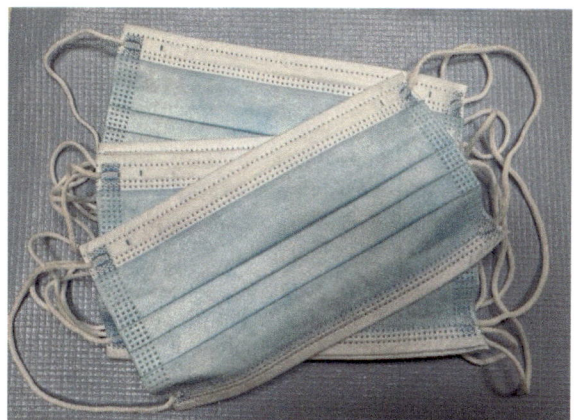

Fig. 7.6 N95 mask. (Photo taken by author)

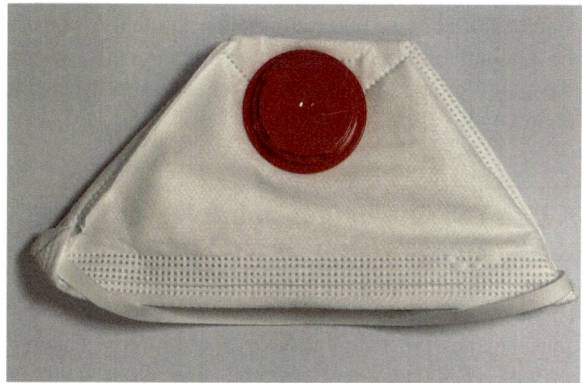

FFP2 respirators availability and insufficient training on how to perform a fit check (Fig. 7.6).

7.6.7   How to Check the User Seal

Use these steps to carry out a user seal check:

1. *Checking the positive pressure user seal*: Gently release your breath while obstructing the airflow from the respirator. A successful check occurs when the respirator experiences a little amount of pressure without leaking.
2. *Check the negative pressure user seal* by quickly inhaling while obstructing the airways leading to the facepiece. The facepiece collapsing slightly under the negative pressure indicates a successful check.

Table 7.7 Difference between qualitative and quantitative fit testing

Qualitative fit testing	For this test you need a trained person and the necessary equipment which consists of a hood, nebulizer, and bitter/sweet solution.	This test is not accurate as it is subjective to the user to taste bitter/sweet and detecting leakage. It is not as accurate as the quantitative fit test
Quantitative fit testing	For this test you need highly trained personnel and the equipment	This test is highly accurate; however, the equipment is considerably expensive when compared to the qualitative equipment.

You should perform a user seal check every time you put on your N95 respirator to ensure you achieve an adequate seal [24].

7.6.7.1 Qualitative and Quantitative Fit Testing

Fit testing is carried out to determine the brand, model, and size of respirator that fits the user.

When selecting a respirator, it is important to consider not only whether it passes the qualitative or quantitative fit testing, but also whether it is comfortable and easy to use. Prolonged use of a respirator can cause headaches, skin irritation, stress, and anxiety [25] (Table 7.7).

7.7 The Challenges of Implementing Transmission-Based Precautions

There are various challenges when trying to implement transmission-based precautions, such as the availability of single rooms. This major challenge for healthcare institutions is trying to isolate all infective cases in single rooms. In the hospital where I work, if single rooms are not available, we try to cohort patients together with the same organism, and on an everyday basis, we review the single rooms to vacate them if not needed anymore.

Another challenge is the persistent colonization of multidrug-resistant organisms, which makes it more difficult to have single rooms available for other patients.

Another factor that is increasing pressure on the isolation of patients, especially MDROs, is that these organisms are becoming more resistant and becoming pan resistant; furthermore, novel mechanisms of resistance are emerging in healthcare institutions.

Another challenge is to implement these precautions; healthcare facilities need more human resources to take care of such patients.

7.8 Conclusion

When standard precautions are not sufficient to prevent the spread of illnesses in healthcare settings, transmission-based precautions play a crucial role in preventing infection. Health care facilities can reduce the risk of healthcare-associated infections (HAIs) greatly by customizing infection control procedures to the individual routes of transmission, whether through touch, droplet, or airborne particles.

Continuous education, training, and adherence to these precautions will remain crucial to safeguard patients and healthcare personnel as healthcare environments change over time, particularly in response to newly developing infectious diseases such as the COVID-19 pandemic.

Combining transmission-based measures with standard precautions creates a complete framework for infection prevention and control that improves outcomes for all parties involved and ensures safer healthcare settings.

References

1. Mayo Clinic. Infectious diseases-Infectious diseases—Symptoms & causes—[Internet]. Mayo Clinic. 2022 [cited 2024 Sep 9]. Available from: https://www.mayoclinic.org/diseases-conditions/infectious-diseases/symptoms-causes/syc-20351173).
2. CDC. Isolation precautions [Internet]. Centers for disease control and prevention. 2019. Available from: https://www.cdc.gov/infectioncontrol/guidelines/isolation/index.html
3. World Health Organization. Infectious diseases. World Health Organization [Internet]. 2016 Jan 22; Available from: https://www.who.int/topics/infectious_diseases/en/. Last accessed 27 July 2024.
4. World Health Organization. Transmission-based precautions for the prevention and control of infections: aide-memoire [Internet]. www.who.int. 2022. Available from: https://www.who.int/publications/i/item/WHO-UHL-IHS-IPC-2022.2.
5. World Health Organization. Global technical consultation report on proposed terminology for pathogens that transmit through the air. World Health Organization; 2024. https://iris.who.int/handle/10665/376496
6. CDC. About ESBL-producing Enterobacterales [Internet]. ESBL-producing Enterobacterales; 2024. Available from: https://www.cdc.gov/esbl-producing-enterobacterales/about/index.html
7. CDC. Clinical overview of tuberculosis disease [internet]. Tuberculosis (TB); 2024. Available from: https://www.cdc.gov/tb/hcp/clinical-overview/tuberculosis-disease.html
8. National Infection Prevention and Control Manual: Transmission Based Precautions definitions [Internet]. Scot.nhs.uk. 2024 [cited 2024 Sep 3]. Available from: https://www.nipcm.hps.scot.nhs.uk/resources/evidence-and-research/transmission-based-precautions-definitions/
9. CDC. Transmission-based precautions [internet]. Infect Control. 2024; Available from: https://www.cdc.gov/infection-control/hcp/basics/transmission-basedprecautions.html?CDC_AAref_Val=https://www.cdc.gov/infectioncontrol/basics/transmission-based-precautions.html
10. NHS England» Glossary of terms [Internet]. www.england.nhs.uk. Available from: https://www.england.nhs.uk/national-infection-prevention-and-control-manual-nipcm-for-england/glossary-of-terms/
11. National Health and Medical Research Council. Australian Guidelines for the Prevention and Control of Infection in healthcare [Internet]. 2019. Available from: https://www.nhmrc.gov.au/sites/default/files/documents/infection-control-guidelines-feb2020.pdf

12. LIM Wei Ling, Wilina et al Recommendations on Implementing Isolation Precautions in Hospital Settings Jointly prepared by Scientific Committee on Infection Control, Infection Control Branch, Centre for Health Protection, Department of Health and Task Force on Infection Control, Hospital Authority [Internet]. 2019. Available from: https://www.chp.gov.hk/files/pdf/recommendations_on_implementing_isolation_precautions_in_hospital_settings.pdf

13. Health Protection Surveillance Centre. Acute Hospital Infection Prevention and Control Precautions for Possible or Confirmed COVID-19 in a Pandemic Setting [Internet]. Available from: https://www.hpsc.ie/a-z/respiratory/coronavirus/novel-coronavirus/guidance/guidanceforhealthcareworkers/acutehospitalsguidance/InfectionPreventionandControlPrecautionsforAcuteSettings.pdf

14. World Health Organization. Infection prevention and control of epidemic- and pandemic-prone acute respiratory infections in health care. World Health Organization; 2014. https://iris.who.int/handle/10665/112656

15. CDC. I. Review of scientific data regarding transmission of infectious agents in healthcare settings [internet]. Infection Control; 2024. [cited 2024 Sep 4]. Available from: https://www.cdc.gov/infection-control/hcp/isolation-precautions/scientific-review.html

16. National Health Service. NHS England» National Infection Prevention and Control [Internet]. www.england.nhs.uk. 2022. Available from: https://www.england.nhs.uk/publication/national-infection-prevention-and-control/

17. CDC. About viral hemorrhagic fevers [internet]. Viral Hemorrhagic Fevers (VHFs); 2024. Available from: https://www.cdc.gov/viral-hemorrhagic-fevers/about/index.html

18. National Services Scotland Aerosol-generating procedures: current situation for Scotland [Internet]. 2023 [cited 2024 Sep 8]. Available from: https://www.nipcm.hps.scot.nhs.uk/media/2088/2023-02-10-agp-sbar-v12.pdf

19. Klompas M, Baker M, Rhee C. What is an aerosol-generating procedure? JAMA Surg. 2021;156(2):113.

20. UK IPC Cell Classification: Official Publication approval reference: C1632 A rapid review of aerosol generating procedures (AGPs) [Internet]. Available from: https://www.england.nhs.uk/wp-content/uploads/2022/04/C1632_rapid-review-of-aerosol-generating-procedures.pdf

21. World Health Organization. Infection prevention and control in the context of COVID-19: a guideline, 21 December 2023. World Health Organization; 2023. https://iris.who.int/handle/10665/375200

22. Murongazvombo AS, Jones RS, Rayment M, Mughal N, Azadian B, Donaldson H, et al. Association between SARS-CoV-2 exposure and antibody status among healthcare workers in two London hospitals: a cross-sectional study. Infect Prevent Pract. 2021;3(3):100157.

23. Regli A, Sommerfield A, von Ungern-Sternberg BS. The role of fit testing N95/FFP2/FFP3 masks: a narrative review. Anaesthesia. 2020;76(1)

24. Centers for Disease Control and Prevention. Respirator fit testing. 2022.; Available from: https://www.cdc.gov/niosh/npptl/topics/respirators/disp_part/respsource3fittest.html.

25. Peters MD. N95 respirators for health care workers: the importance of fit, comfort, and usability. Med J Australia. 2022;217(2):83–4.

The Standard Precautions and Behavior About Transmission-Based Precautions Isolation Techniques and Room Placement

8

Maria Gabriela Festa

8.1 Introduction

Infection prevention and control is a practical, evidence-based approach to preventing patients and healthcare workers (HCWs) from contracting preventable infections. Effective Infection Prevention and Control (IPC) programs require targeted and consistent interventions at all levels of the healthcare system (decision-makers, facility managers, HCWs, and those accessing services). Any failure in this system can cause harm and prevent the service from providing quality healthcare.

In a healthcare setting, infection prevention is a key priority to protect the health of patients, HCWs and the community. There are two levels of precautions recommended to prevent the spread of pathogenic microorganisms in healthcare settings: Standard Precautions (SP) and Transmission-Based Precautions.

Every healthcare worker in the context of their activity must avoid spreading microorganisms that can potentially pose a danger to themselves and others (patients, caregivers, visitors, and colleagues). This risk can be prevented through the application of simple and effective behaviors such as those indicated in Standard Precautions and Transmission-Based Precautions. Unfortunately, there is still a poor adherence to these measures and the main difficulties are in identifying when and how they should be applied. It is necessary to share the criteria for their application and increase awareness of the importance of precautions among HCWs through training and promotion of good practices.

Let's analyze each of these categories and their impact on clinical practice.

M. G. Festa (✉)
ASST Spedali Civili di Brescia—Children's Hospital, Brescia, Italy
e-mail: gabriela.festa@asst-spedalicivili.it

© The Author(s), under exclusive license to Springer Nature Switzerland AG 2025
B. Oomen, S. Gastaldi (eds.), *Principles of Nursing Infection Prevention Control*,
Principles of Specialty Nursing, https://doi.org/10.1007/978-3-031-84469-0_8

8.2 Standard Precautions: The First Line of Defense Against Infections

Standard precautions aim to protect both HCWs and patients by reducing the risk of transmission of microorganisms from both recognized and unrecognized sources. They are the minimum standard of IPC practices that should be used by all healthcare workers, during the care of all patients, at all times, in all settings. When applied consistently, standard precautions can prevent the transmission of microorganisms between patients, HCWs, and the environment [1].

They are therefore a set of practices designed to prevent the transmission of infections in healthcare settings, home care, and nursing homes. They must be adopted for every patient, regardless of diagnosis or health status.

Compared to the measures that we all know, which refer to the recommendations of the CDC [2], in June 2022 the WHO [3] produced a five-page memo to remember the key elements and advice for implementing standard precautions. Some interesting additions are proposed in this memo such as the following:

- risk assessment,
- personal protective equipment (respirators such as N95, FFP2),
- aseptic technique, and
- decontamination and reprocessing of reusable patient care items and equipment

This document provides guidance directed at organizations, focusing on structural and organizational aspects essential for effective implementation, as well as key elements for daily practice. The first set of recommendations is intended for decision-makers, emphasizing the need to establish the appropriate infrastructure, organizational frameworks, and resources to enable frontline workers to apply these measures. The second set is tailored to individual operators, outlining behaviors and best practices necessary for effective risk prevention.

8.2.1 Key Elements and Guidance for the Implementation Standard Precautions

The main measures included in these precautions are aimed to the "decision-makers" who must put the structure, organizational model, and resources in conditions so that these measures can be applied by operators. We are therefore talking about health policy.

Health Policy
- Promote a climate of safety.
- Develop policies that facilitate the implementation of IPC practice.
- Provide resources for IPC programs and implementation of standard precautions.

8.2.2 Standard Precautions in Continuous Evolution

As new infection control challenges arise, guideline developers must determine if any content of SP needs to be changed (e.g., hand hygiene materials or methods). SP are the gold standard and should be practiced for every patient and by every HCW in the healthcare setting [4].

The concept is simple: SP are what should be done at all times and should be present in all healthcare settings at all times, to minimize the risk of acquiring infections. Effectively translating this into clear, concise, and accurate language is not easy.

In an effort to present an easy-to-understand summary of SP, the following definition is proposed: SP are designed to prevent cross-transmission and infection when receiving healthcare, when providing healthcare, or when simply present in a healthcare setting. They are a minimum set of actions that should be practiced at all times in every healthcare setting and should be used at all times for every healthcare procedure.

SP for the prevention and control of infections consist of the following practices:

- Risk assessment
- Hand hygiene
- Respiratory hygiene and cough etiquette
- Patient placement
- Personal protective equipment (PPE)
- Aseptic technique
- Safe injections and sharps injury prevention
- Decontamination and reprocessing of reusable patient care items and equipment
- Environment and environmental cleaning

8.2.2.1 Risk Assessment

Risk assessment should be performed always before any interaction with the patient and adopt all those measures and barriers useful for the protection of operators and patients.

This assessment is independent from the knowledge of microbiology or infectious diseases, but there are elements to consider in the choice of protective measures:

- The procedure to be performed (e.g., blood sampling, insertion of a bladder catheter)
- Any signs and symptoms of the patient (e.g., fever, cough, diarrhea)
- The structural conditions (e.g., single room, emergency room environment)
- The skills of the operator (e.g., newly hire staff, staff in training, new procedure)

Organizations must train operators in a model of application of standard precautions through the "risk assessment at the point of care."

HCWs should:

- assess the risk of exposure to blood and body fluids, secretions/excretions, splashes and/or sprays, or contaminated surfaces before any healthcare activity [3–5] and make it routine.
- select appropriate actions to reduce the risk of exposure to infectious agents;
- ask themselves before any interaction with the patient:
  - Do I need protection for what I am about to do because there is a risk of exposure to blood and body fluids, secretions, excretions, splashes, and/or sprays?
  - Do I need protection for what I am about to do because the patient has symptoms of an undiagnosed infection?
  - Do I need protection for what I am about to do because the patient has symptoms of an undiagnosed infection that requires transmission-based precautions?
  - Do I need protection for what I am about to do because the patient has a known infection that requires transmission-based precautions?

For each affirmative answer to these key questions, it is necessary to identify those standard precaution measures necessary to prevent contamination during direct contact and the measures to be adopted in the event of indirect contamination.

8.2.2.2 Hand Hygiene: The Gesture That Saves Lives

Hand hygiene is the main measure for preventing infections and the spread of multiresistant germs, but at the same time, it is one of the most neglected practices even though the indications contained in the international guidelines of the WHO are simple and easy to perform.

To overcome this difficulty and to make the WHO indications applicable, "the concept of the five moments of hand hygiene" was developed. This conceptual model transforms the indications for hand hygiene into five moments of hand hygiene that are carried out in and around a space: the patient point of patient care.

WHO has published in the guidelines and manuals on hand hygiene the description of the conceptual model that has been summarized in the poster that we all know. These Guidelines are intended to be implemented in any situation where healthcare is provided to a patient or a specific group of a population. Therefore, this concept applies to all environments where healthcare is provided on a permanent or occasional basis, such as home care [5].

The poster "Your 5 moments for hand hygiene," represents one of the reminders in the workplace, key tools to signal and remind operators of the importance of good practices, therefore they must be understood and placed at key points of the health activity.

All the elements represented are structured around a key word: "Touch." We speak of contact when, during care and assistance activities, the operators' hands can touch:

- the patient's intact skin or personal effects,
- the patient's mucous membranes or non-intact skin,
- inserted invasive medical devices,
- the patient's body fluids,
- medical or electromedical devices,
- inanimate environmental surfaces around the patient.

Hands should be washed with soap and water when visibly soiled and after using the toilet. Duration of the entire procedure: 40–60 s.

Handrubbing with an alcohol-based hand rub (ABHR) is the preferred method for hand cleansing in the healthcare setting when hands are not visibly soiled. ABHRs should be applied to dry hands. Duration of the entire procedure: 20–30 s.

Updated hand hygiene guidelines were published in February 2023 [6]; the recommendations are intended for acute care hospitals but can be adapted to all hospitals and home care facilities. This expert guidance document is sponsored by the Society for Healthcare Epidemiology (SHEA) in collaboration with other leading scientific societies and organizations interested in healthcare security.

The recommendations are divided into "essential practices," which should be adopted by all acute care hospitals, and "additional practices," which are useful to consider in facilities or patient groups where HAIs have not been effectively controlled after the implementation of essential practices (Table 8.1).

To improve hand hygiene practice, changing the behaviors is essential; multimodal strategies are the most effective approach to improve hand hygiene.

Adherence to hand hygiene is a priority for the facility and requires appropriate leadership, administrative support, and available economic resources.

For all these reasons, it is important to actively participate in training programs started in your facility and to be aware of how easily and quickly hands become contaminated during care activities.

8.2.2.3 Respiratory Hygiene and Cough Etiquette: A Response to Infectious Emergencies

There is very little published evidence examining cough/respiratory hygiene etiquette.

Much of the available material is limited to professional opinion and is based on the 2007 CDC isolation guidelines [2].

Cough/respiratory hygiene etiquette can be defined as source control measures aimed at

Table 8.1 Seven essential hand hygiene practices (according to SHEA, 2022)

Promote the maintenance of healthy hand skin and fingernails.
Select appropriate products.
Ensure the accessibility of hand hygiene supplies.
Ensure appropriate glove use to reduce hand and environmental contamination.
Take steps to reduce environmental contamination associated with sinks and sink drains.
Monitor adherence to hand hygiene.
Provide timely and meaningful feedback to enhance a culture of safety.

containing respiratory secretions in order to limit transmission of respiratory pathogens spread by droplets or airways, particularly during seasonal outbreaks of viral respiratory tract infections in the community.

To prevent the spread of respiratory viruses, appropriate measures must be taken at the point of reception of a patient (e.g., triage, outpatient clinic, doctor's office) with respiratory signs and symptoms. The two key actions are hand hygiene and cough etiquette, which must be adopted when the person presents signs and symptoms of infection such as cough, fever, or cold symptoms.

The following measures to contain respiratory secretions are also recommended for all individuals with signs and symptoms of respiratory infection. These measures apply to any person with signs of illness including cough, congestion, runny nose, or increased production of respiratory secretions:

- post posters at the entrance of healthcare facilities to provide guidance on what to do if you have respiratory signs and symptoms;
- teach people with respiratory symptoms about respiratory hygiene/cough etiquette;
- place supplies of tissues available in common areas (e.g., waiting rooms), hand hygiene products, masks, and no-touch waste containers in waiting areas;
- use tissues or masks when coughing, such as into your sleeve or shoulder or when turning your head, to contain respiratory secretions and promptly dispose of used tissues and perform hand hygiene immediately afterwards;
- put a mask on people with coughs, providing that it is clinically safe to do so and tolerated by the patient;
- Maintain a spatial separation of at least 1 m between patients with symptoms of acute respiratory infection (manifested by cough, dyspnea, and fever) and those without symptoms.

8.2.2.4 Patient Placement: Assessment for Infection Risk

Standard Precautions (SP) also emphasize the principle of source control, which involves the prompt identification of patients with communicable diseases and their appropriate placement. At triage—the initial assessment of a patient's symptoms and reason for admission to the healthcare facility—source control includes the rapid recognition of symptoms of active infection and the spatial separation of patients with communicable diseases from others.

Patients showing symptoms of acute infections, such as cough, fever, vomiting, diarrhea, runny nose, rash, or conjunctivitis, should be assigned to designated waiting areas separate from other patients. Physical barriers should be used to separate infectious patients, particularly those with respiratory symptoms, from susceptible individuals or other patients. Patients suspected or confirmed to have airborne infections should be placed directly in a negative pressure room. Those with acute diarrheal illness should be directed to an examining room equipped with a dedicated bathroom or commode.

Infection risk should be promptly assessed upon the patient's arrival in the care area—such as an emergency department, inpatient unit, outpatient clinic, or nursing home—and continuously reassessed during their stay. This evaluation should inform decisions on patient placement based on clinical and care needs. Patients who may pose a cross-infection risk include those with diarrhea, vomiting, unexplained rashes, fever, or respiratory symptoms; those known to have previously tested positive for a multidrug-resistant organism (MDRO), such as carbapenemase-producing Enterobacteriaceae (CPE); and individuals recently admitted to a hospital abroad or with a known epidemiological link to an MDRO carrier.

While single-room accommodations are optimal for infection control, they may not always be available in sufficient numbers in healthcare settings. Single rooms should be prioritized for patients who pose a risk of transmission to others, such as those who contaminate their environment or have symptoms of a communicable infection [3].

8.2.2.5 Personal Protective Equipment: The Protective Shield

Before undertaking any procedure, staff should assess any likely exposure to blood and/or other body fluids, non-intact skin or mucous membranes and wear Personal Protective Equipment (PPE) that adequately protects against the risks associated with the procedure.

The principles of PPE use set out below are important to ensure that PPE is used correctly to ensure the safety of patients and staff. Avoiding excessive or inappropriate use of PPE is a key principle that ensures this is risk-based and minimizes its environmental impact. Where appropriate, the environmental impact of sustainable or reusable PPE options compared to single-use PPE should be considered, adhering to the principles below [2].

All PPE should be:

- placed close to the point of use. PPE for HCWs providing care in the community and home care workers should be transported in a clean container;
- stored to prevent contamination in a clean, dry area until use (observe expiry dates);
- single use, unless otherwise specified by the manufacturer;
- changed immediately after each patient and/or after completing a procedure or task disposed of after use in the appropriate waste stream, e.g., household waste, offensive (noninfectious) or clinical waste;
- disposed of if damaged or contaminated.

NB. Reusable PPE, such as goggles/face shields/visors, should be decontaminated after each use in accordance with the manufacturer's instructions.

Gloves must be:

- worn when exposure to blood and/or other body fluids, non-intact skin or mucous membranes is anticipated or likely;
- changed immediately after each patient and/or after completing a procedure/task even on the same patient, and after performing hand hygiene;
- changed if a perforation or puncture is suspected
- appropriate for use, fit for purpose and well-fitting

- never decontaminated with ABHR or soap between uses
- low risk of causing sensitization to the wearer
- appropriate for the tasks performed, taking into account the substances handled, the type and duration of contact, the size and comfort of the gloves, as well as the task and the requirements for strength and sensitivity of the gloves.

Sterile gloves must be worn:

- when sterility is required in an operating room and
- for certain aseptic techniques, such as the insertion of central venous catheters, insertion of peripherally inserted central catheters, insertion of pulmonary artery catheters, and spinal, epidural, and caudal procedures

NB: Double gloving is NOT recommended for routine clinical care. However, it may be necessary for certain procedures with exposure, such as orthopedic and gynecological operations, when attending major traumatic incidents or as part of additional precautions for the management of high-risk infectious diseases.

NB: Gloves are NOT required for administrative tasks in close proximity to the patient, such as using the telephone, using a computer or tablet, writing in the patient record; administering oral medications; serving meals.

Gowns or fluid-resistant suits should be:

- worn when there is a risk of extensive splashing of blood and/or body fluids, e.g., operating room, ICU
- worn when a disposable apron does not provide adequate coverage for the procedure or task being performed
- changed between patients and removed immediately after completing a sterile procedure or task when sterility is required in an operating room and for certain aseptic techniques, e.g., insertion of central venous catheters, insertion of peripherally inserted central catheters, insertion of pulmonary artery catheters, and spinal, epidural, and caudal procedures.

Medical masks are required:

- as a means of source control, for example, to protect the patient from the wearer during sterile procedures such as surgery,
- to protect the wearer when there is a risk of splashes or sprays of blood, body fluids, secretions, or excretions on the respiratory mucosa;
- as an element of PPE for droplet precautions

Medical mask should be:

- worn (with eye protection) if a full face shield is not available and blood, body fluids, secretions or excretions are expected or likely to be splashed or sprayed onto the respiratory mucosa (nose and mouth) (type IIR);

- worn to protect patients from the operator as a source of infection, for example when performing surgical or epidural procedures or inserting a central vascular catheter (CVC);
- tight-fitting and fit for purpose, completely covering the mouth and nose (manufacturer's instructions should be followed to ensure effective fit and protection)

Medical mask should be removed or changed:

- at the end of a procedure/task
- if the integrity of the mask is compromised, for example, due to moisture accumulation after prolonged use or severe contamination with blood or body fluids
- in accordance with the manufacturer's specific instructions.

Eye or face protection (including full face shields). HCWs should:

- wear eye protection (face shield, goggles) or a visor to protect the mucous membranes of the eyes during activities that may generate splashes or sprays of blood, body fluids, secretions, and excretions;
- ensure that eyewear fits over and around the eyes or personal prescription lenses;
- regular corrective glasses are not considered eye protection
- ensure that a visor covers the forehead, extends under the chin, and wraps around the side of the face: note that visors are more comfortable to wear with glasses.

Head Covering

Head covering is not routinely required in clinical areas unless it is part of the operating theatre attire or to prevent contamination of the environment, such as in clean rooms.

Head covering should be:

- worn in the operating theatre and clean rooms, for example in the central decontamination unit
- well-fitting and completely covering the hair
- changed or disposed of between clinical procedures/lists or tasks and if contaminated with blood and/or body fluids
- removed before leaving the operating theatre or clean room
- individuals with facial hair must also cover this in areas where headwear is required (e.g., wear a snood)

NB: Head coverings worn for religious reasons, such as turbans, kippot veils, scarves, should not compromise patient and healthcare worker safety. They should be washed and/or changed daily or immediately if contaminated.

8.2.2.6 Aseptic Technique

The aseptic technique is an essential nursing and medical skill in reducing healthcare-associated infections. It aims to prevent the transfer of microorganisms from the HCWs, the procedure equipment or from the immediate environment to the patient [7].

An aseptic technique is used during a medical procedure that enters the body site, usually by puncturing the skin (inserting indwelling devices, e.g., IV cannulas, CVC catheters), inserting instruments into a body cavity (e.g., endoscopy), or cutting the skin in a surgical procedure. In addition, the aseptic technique is also used to maintain indwelling devices and manage wound dressing.

Aseptic technique, when performed correctly will:

- minimize contamination of key sites,
- protect patients from their own pathogenic microorganisms that may cause infection,
- reduce the transmission of microorganisms, and
- maintain the sterility of equipment and key parts used for aseptic procedures

HCWs should:

- use sterile items and equipment for all aseptic procedures;
- use aseptic technique for insertion and maintenance of all invasive devices and aseptic/clean clinical procedures for surgical procedures, wound dressing, and similar, to prevent infections.

8.2.2.7 Safe Injections and Sharps Injury Prevention

Unsafe injection practices are associated with the transmission and outbreaks of blood-borne viruses (HIV, Hepatitis B, and C). Therefore, all staff must receive education and training in safe injection practices. In addition, the following measures must be taken to achieve safe injection practices in healthcare facilities [8]:

- Prepare all injections in a dedicated, clean, organized area, as it is vital in preventing contamination with microorganisms. The area should meet the essential requirements for safe injection preparation. The area must not be contaminated with blood and/or body fluids. Any contaminated items, including blood samples, must not be brought to this room or area.
- Healthcare workers must always perform hand hygiene before preparing injections and before and after giving an injection.
- Carefully inspect the packaging before opening it and discard the syringe and needle if it has been damaged or moist.
- Always use a sterile and safety-engineered syringes and needle from a new and sealed package. If the sterility of the pack is compromised (e.g., a break in sterile packaging), use a new pack of undamaged syringes.
- Never reuse needles or syringes, as they are single-use items only.
- Use single-dose vials where feasible.
- Each medication/vaccine should be administered aseptically and separately.
- Clean skin if it is visibly dirty and then disinfect skin by applying 60–70% alcohol isopropyl alcohol (± 2% chlorhexidine) solution on the skin till it is dry.

There is a potential risk of blood-borne virus transmission from significant occupational exposure. Therefore, staff must understand the actions they should take when a significant occupational exposure incident occurs.

The injured healthcare worker should report sharp injuries and other significant exposure to blood and body fluids to the line manager or occupational health.

There is a legal requirement to report all sharps injuries and near misses to line managers/employers.

8.2.2.8 Decontamination and Reprocessing of Reusable Patient Care Items and Equipment

Care equipment is easily contaminated with blood, other body fluids, secretions, excretions, and infectious agents. Consequently, it is easy to transfer infectious agents from communal care equipment during care delivery.

Care equipment is classified as either:

- single use: equipment which is used once on a single patient then discarded. This equipment must never be reused. The packaging will carry the symbol of the number two in a circle with a diagonal cross
- single patient use: equipment which can be reused on the same patient and may require decontamination in-between use such as nebulizer masks
- reusable invasive equipment: used once then decontaminated, e.g., surgical instruments and solid-state reusable equipment, flexible endoscopes, and transducers
- reusable noninvasive equipment: reused on more than one patient following decontamination between each use, e.g., commode, patient transfer trolley.

NB: Needles and syringes are single-use devices; they should never be used more than once or reused to draw up additional medication. Never administer medications from a single-dose vial or intravenous (IV) bag to multiple patients.

HCWs should:

- handle equipment contaminated with blood, body fluids, secretions, and excretions in a manner that prevents exposure of skin and mucous membranes, contamination of clothing and transfer of pathogens to other patients or the environment;
- clean and disinfect (or sterilize, depending on the type and use of patient care equipment) reusable equipment before use with other patients;
- dispose of single-use devices after each use;
- clean and disinfect or sterilize reusable equipment/devices according to the manufacturer's instructions, national or international standards, using efficient methods and according to the intended use.

8.2.2.9 Environment and Environmental Cleaning

Environmental cleaning is part of SP, which should be applied to all patients in all healthcare facilities. It is important to implement environmental cleaning programmes as part of facility-wide IPC programmes. Wherever possible, for example, during staff training and education, consider creating synergies and highlighting the relationship between environmental cleaning and hand hygiene activities in preventing environmental transmission of HAIs [9].

Contaminated hands or gloves will also continue to spread microorganisms around the environment.

HCWs should:

- clean and disinfect patient care areas at least once a day, paying particular attention to frequently touched surfaces.
- deal with spills of blood and body fluid/substance as soon as possible, in accordance with local protocols.

8.3   Transmission-Based Precautions and Room Placement

Transmission-based precautions (TBP) are used in addition to standard precautions for patients with known or suspected infection or colonization with transmissible and/or epidemiologically significant pathogens. The type of transmission-based precautions assigned to a patient depends on the route of transmission of the microorganism [2]:

- contact,
- droplet, or
- airborne transmission

TBP should be started as soon as a patient presents with symptoms (e.g., fever, new cough, vomiting, diarrhea). There is no need to wait for test results.

8.3.1   Contact Precautions

Contact Precautions are intended to prevent transmission of infectious agents, including epidemiologically important microorganisms, which are spread by direct or indirect contact with the patient or the patient's environment.

- Direct contact transmission involves both a direct body-surface-to-body-surface contact and physical transfer of microorganisms between an infected or colonized person and a susceptible host.
- Indirect contact transmission involves contact of a susceptible host with a contaminated intermediate object (e.g., contaminated hands) that carries and transfers the microorganisms.

Contact Precautions also apply where the presence of excessive wound drainage, fecal incontinence, or other discharges from the body suggest an increased potential for extensive environmental contamination and risk of transmission.

A single-patient room is preferred for patients who require Contact Precautions. When a single room is not available, it is recommended that other patient accommodation options be considered with an appropriate risk assessment (e.g., cohorting). In multi-patient rooms, ≥1 m (≥3 feet) spatial separation between beds is advised to reduce the opportunities for inadvertent sharing of items between the infected/colonized patient and other patients. Healthcare personnel caring for patients on contact precautions wear a gown and gloves for all interactions that may involve contact with the patient or potentially contaminated areas in the patient's environment. Donning PPE upon room entry and discarding before exiting the patient room is done to contain pathogens, especially those that have been implicated in transmission through environmental contamination (e.g., VRE, *C. difficile, noroviruses* and other intestinal tract pathogens; RSV)

8.3.2   Droplet Precautions

Droplet transmission is the spread of an infectious agent caused by the dissemination of droplets. Droplets are primarily generated from an infected (source) person during coughing, sneezing, and talking. Transmission occurs when these droplets that contain microorganisms are propelled (usually <1 m) through the air and deposited on the conjunctivae, mouth, nasal, throat or pharynx mucosa of another person. Most of the volume (>99%) comprises large droplets that travel short distances (<1 m) and do not remain suspended in the air. Thus, special air handling and ventilation are not required to prevent droplet transmission.

A single patient room is preferred for patients who require droplet precautions. When a single-patient room is not available, consultation with infection control personnel is recommended to assess the various risks associated with other patient placement options (e.g., cohorting, keeping the patient with an existing roommate). Spatial separation of ≥ 1 m and drawing the curtain between patient beds is especially important for patients in multi-bed rooms with infections transmitted by the droplet route. Healthcare personnel wear a mask (a respirator is not necessary) for close contact with infectious patient; the mask is generally donned upon room entry.

Patients on droplet precautions who must be transported outside of the room should wear a mask if tolerated and follow respiratory hygiene/cough etiquette.

8.3.3   Airborne Precautions

Airborne precautions prevent transmission of infectious agents that remain infectious over long distances when suspended in the air, for example, rubeola virus (measles), varicella virus (chickenpox), *M. tuberculosis*, and possibly SARS-CoV.

The preferred placement for patients who require airborne precautions is in an airborne infection isolation room (AIIR). An AIIR is a single-patient room that is equipped with special air handling and ventilation capacity (i.e., monitored negative pressure relative to the surrounding area, 12 air exchanges per hour for new construction and renovation, and 6 air exchanges per hour for existing facilities, air exhausted directly to the outside or recirculated through HEPA filtration before return). Some states require the availability of such rooms in hospitals, emergency departments, and nursing homes that care for patients with *M. tuberculosis*.

A respiratory protection program that includes education about use of respirators, fit-testing, and user seal checks is required in any facility with AIIRs. In settings where Airborne Precautions cannot be implemented due to limited engineering resources, masking the patient, placing the patient in a private room (e.g., office examination room or single room) with the door closed, and providing N95 or higher level respirators or masks if respirators are not available for healthcare personnel will reduce the likelihood of airborne transmission until the patient is either transferred to a facility with an AIIR or returned to the home environment, as deemed medically appropriate.

Healthcare personnel caring for patients on airborne precautions wear a mask NH95 or respirator, depending on the disease-specific recommendations, that is donned prior to room entry.

Whenever possible, nonimmune HCWs should not care for patients with vaccine-preventable airborne diseases (e.g., measles, chickenpox, and smallpox).

8.3.4 Factors to Consider When Placing Patients in Isolation Rooms

One important factor is the type of isolation required, e.g. patients requiring airborne isolation should be placed in a negative-pressure room with a HEPA filter. Patients requiring droplet isolation should be placed in a private room or in a cohort with other patients with the same infection. Patients requiring contact isolation can be placed in a private room or in a cohort with other patients with the same infection.

Another factor to be considered is the patient's condition: Patients who are severely ill or immunocompromised may require more stringent isolation measures.

Also, availability of isolation rooms should be considered because the number and type of isolation rooms available in the facility will influence room placement decisions.

Additional considerations for isolation and room placement include:

- PPE—HCWs must wear appropriate PPE when entering isolation rooms to protect themselves and prevent the spread of infection.
- Environmental cleaning and disinfection—isolation rooms must be thoroughly cleaned and disinfected after each patient to prevent the transmission of pathogens.

- Ventilation—proper ventilation is essential in isolation rooms, especially for airborne diseases.
- Staff training—HCWs must be trained on isolation techniques and room placement procedures to ensure their effectiveness.

8.4   Conclusion

Standard Precautions and Transmission-Based Precautions are essential tools in the fight against healthcare-associated infections and in protecting public health. Strict application of these measures not only helps safeguard patients and HCWs but is also a critical step toward reducing infections and improving the overall quality of care. Investing in education and awareness of these practices is essential to ensuring safe and effective healthcare.

While SP are the basic practices used consistently for all patients, Transmission-Based Precautions are additional measures used when SP alone may not be sufficient to prevent transmission.

It is critical that HCWs are adequately trained and that practices are continually reviewed and updated based on the latest evidence.

Disclosure   Maria Gabriela Festa declares no relevant financial relationships with ineligible companies.

References

1. World Health Organization. Global strategy on infection prevention and control. Accessed 27 July 2024; 2023.
2. Siegel JD, Rhinehart E, Jackson M, Chiarello L, Health Care Infection Control Practices Advisory Committee. Guideline for isolation precautions: preventing transmission of infectious agents in health care settings. Am J Infect Control. 2007;35(10 Suppl 2):S65–S164. https://doi.org/10.1016/j.ajic.2007.10.007. PMID: 18068815; PMCID: PMC7119119
3. World Health Organization. Standard precautions for the prevention and control of infections: aide-memoire, Technical document. Accessed 13 July 2024; 2022.
4. Curran ET. Standard precautions: what is meant and what is not. J Hosp Infect. 90(1):10–1.
5. WHO. WHO guidelines on hand hygiene in health care. Geneva: World Health Organization; 2009.
6. Glowicz JB, Landon E, Sickbert-Bennett EE, Aiello AE, deKay K, Hoffmann KK, Maragakis L, Olmsted RN, Polgreen PM, Trexler PA, VanAmringe MA, Wood AR, Yokoe D, Ellingson KD. SHEA/IDSA/APIC practice recommendation: strategies to prevent healthcare-associated infections through hand hygiene: 2022 update. Infect Control Hosp Epidemiol. 2023;44(3):355–76. https://doi.org/10.1017/ice.2022.304. Epub 2023 Feb 8. PMID: 36751708; PMCID: PMC10015275
7. Rowley S. Theory to practice. Aseptic non-touch technique. Nursing Times. 2001;97(7):VI–VIII.

8. WHO guideline on the use of safety-engineered syringes for intramuscular, intradermal and subcutaneous injections in health care settings. 01 January 2016. Available from: https://www.who.int/publications/i/item/9789241549820

9. CDC, ICAN. Best practices for environmental cleaning in healthcare facilities in resource-limited settings. Atlanta: Centers for Disease Control and Prevention; 2019. Available from: https://www.cdc.gov/healthcare-associated-infections/media/pdfs/environmental-cleaning-rls-508.pdf

Personal Protective Equipment (PPE)

9

Tihana Gašpert

9.1 Introduction

Nurses must possess a thorough comprehension of infection prevention and control to safeguard themselves, patients, colleagues, and the public against the spread of infection. Personal protective equipment (PPE), including gloves, aprons and/or gowns, masks, and eye protection, is crucial for infection prevention and control among healthcare professionals, particularly nurses. Effective utilization of PPE necessitates thorough evaluation, comprehension of the appropriateness of different PPE types in different clinical situations, and proper implementation. Gaining a comprehensive understanding of the function of PPE empowers nurses to utilize it effectively and minimize avoidable expenses, all while maintaining the nurse-patient connection as the core focus of care [1].

9.2 Types of Personal Protective Equipment

PPE consists of a gown, gloves, masks, and face shields or goggles. Comprehending the restrictions and correct utilization of PPE is crucial for guaranteeing the implementation of secure procedures [2].

9.2.1 Gloves

Various gloves provide varying levels of requirements for preventing infections [2]. The acceptable quality level (AQL) is a frequently employed criterion for evaluating

T. Gašpert (✉)
University Hospital Rijeka, Rijeka, Croatia

Faculty of Health Sciences, University of Maribor, Maribor, Slovenia

glove safety. A lower Acceptable Quality Level (AQL) indicates a superior glove quality, characterized by less risk of micro-perforation and fewer pinholes in the product. The FDA typically advises a minimum Acceptable Quality Level (AQL) of 1.5 for surgical gloves and 2.5 for medical examination gloves [3].

It is important to wear nonsterile, well-fitting, disposable gloves in the following situations:

• When handling materials that may be infectious or when touching contaminated items and surfaces.
• When there is a chance of direct contact with a patient's blood or other potentially infectious materials, such as body fluids, moist body substances, saliva (during dental procedures), mucous membranes, or damaged skin.

There is a risk of blood exposure at the puncture site during venipuncture or venous access injections. This risk is heightened if the nurse or patient has compromised skin integrity, such as eczema, cracked skin, or dry skin. Additionally, skin conditions like eczema, burns, or skin infections in the patient can also increase the risk of blood exposure.

Replace gloves:

• Between tasks and procedures on the same patient, as well as after coming into contact with material that may contain a significant amount of microorganisms.
• During a procedure if gloves become dirty, torn, or punctured.—After meeting each patient.

Upon completion of treatment and before departing patient-care areas, rapidly remove and dispose of gloves, and immediately engage in hand hygiene.

Gloves do not serve as a substitute for hand hygiene.

Use sterile gloves exclusively for procedures requiring an aseptic technique, such as intravascular infusion and devices.

When administering injections, wearing gloves for regular intradermal, subcutaneous, and intramuscular injections is not recommended, if the nurse's skin is undamaged.

Latex allergy is a severe and potentially fatal illness that impacts 8–12% [4] of individuals who regularly use natural rubber latex gloves. Nurses who have a hypersensitivity to natural rubber latex should avoid any form of interaction with latex-based goods. Nurses who have an allergic reaction should utilize gloves composed of synthetic materials.

Gloves do not offer protection against needle-stick or other puncture injuries caused by sharp objects. Needles, scalpels, and other sharp objects should be handled carefully [4].

9.2.2 Gowns

Gowns are recognized as the second most often utilized kind of PPE, behind gloves. As per the Centers for Disease Control and Prevention's Guideline for Isolation Precautions, nurses should wear isolation gowns to safeguard their arms and other exposed body parts while performing procedures and engaging in patient-care activities that involve potential contact with clothing, blood, bodily fluids, secretions, and excretions. The isolation gowns currently available in the market exhibit different levels of resistance to blood and other biological fluids, which rely on factors such as material type, impermeability, and durability. While certain studies indicate no advantage to the regular utilization of isolation gowns, others indicate that their use is linked to a decreased infection rate [5].

Within the realm of PPE design, there are several unresolved concerns about the design of isolation gowns. These include the following:

- the time and procedure for putting on and taking off clothing;
- the effectiveness of the gown as a barrier, including the quality of the seams and closures;
- the comfort of the clothing in terms of thermal regulation, ease of mobility, and proper sizing and fit [6].

Having access to suitable gowns can effectively hinder the transmission of infection. Medical gowns adhere to the ANSI/AAMI PB70 standards set by the American National Standards Institute (ANSI), the Association of the Advancement of Medical Instrumentation (AAMI), and the Food and Drug Administration (FDA). The ANSI/AAMI PB70 standard categorizes fluid barrier protection into four tiers [7].

The USP 800 recommendations enhance safety by specifying the requirements for gowns when handling dangerous medications. Adhering to recommended protocols for PPE in a suitable environment, whether utilizing aseptic gowns for surgical procedures or nonsterile gowns for potential contact exposure, will guarantee the safety of both healthcare professionals and patients [2, 8].

9.2.3 Masks

Loosely woven cotton masks offer minimal respiratory protection, whereas respirators recognized by the National Institute for Occupational Safety and Health (NIOSH) provide the highest level of protection [9, 10]. An essential aspect of mask protection entails ensuring the masks are fitted correctly [11]. It is necessary to do fit testing for all healthcare personnel who are mandated to use respirators, such as N95 masks [12, 13].

Face masks can be categorized into different groups:

9.2.3.1 Fabric Masks

A cloth face mask is an affordable and commonly constructed protective covering, typically crafted from everyday cotton fabric, designed to be worn over the mouth and nose. Health authorities are mandated to utilize fabric masks for protection when medical masks are not accessible in inventory [14]. It is composed entirely of several types of fabric. Research indicates that fabric masks are less efficient than other masks in protecting against infections. However, they still offer some basic protection. It offers the user protection against airborne pollutants such as pollen and dust particles.

According to laboratory data and the guidance provided by the World Health Organization (WHO), textile masks can be classified into three types:

(a) Cloth mask 1.
(b) Cloth mask 2.
(c) Cloth mask 3.

Fabric mask 1 is equipped with a latex exhalation valve, which demonstrated superior performance compared to the other two fabric masks lacking an exhalation valve. The filtering efficiency of cloth masks 2 and 3 differed depending on the various sizes of PSL (polystyrene latex) particles. Cloth masks 2 and 3 are more prone to being penetrated compared to cloth mask 1. Cloth mask 1 is a highly effective filtering mask that has a conical or tetrahedral shape, making it suitable for use by the public. The mask also consists of three layers, including a hydrophilic inner layer, a filter in the middle layer, and a hydrophobic outer layer. In contrast, cloth masks 2 and 3 feature basic rectangular loops and lack the three-layer structure. Cloth mask 2 consists of two layers, specifically a filter layer and a hydrophobic outer layer. In contrast, cloth mask 3 just comprises a single thin layer. Cloth mask 1 had superior filtering performance and fit compared to the other two masks. Nevertheless, cloth mask 2 exhibited superior performance in comparison to cloth mask. Highly effective fabric face masks should consist of a minimum of three layers, with an inside layer that is capable of absorbing moisture from the wearer's breath (such as cotton) and outside layers that repel moisture (such as polyester) [15].

9.2.3.2 Masks Used for Medical or Surgical Purposes

A Type-IIR medical face mask, which is resistant to fluids, is used to protect against droplets. When worn, it will reduce the spread of large respiratory droplets, protecting from both droplets and the transmission of viruses. When wearing it, the mask protects against droplet transmission within 1–2 m from the infected person. An estimated reduction of at least 80% in danger is calculated [16]. Surgical masks consist of three layers: an inner soft absorbent layer, a middle polypropylene barrier, and an outer hydrophobic surface. This face mask provides effective protection from droplets in a healthcare environment. The design of surgical masks is based on the mode, typically consisting of three-ply (three layers) or four-ply (four layers) configurations. This fabric consists of three layers, with a middle layer made of a melt-blown polymer, often polypropylene, sandwiched between two layers of non-woven cloth. The mask consists of three distinct layers. The outermost layer is designed to reject water droplets, while the middle layer acts as a filter. The inner-most layer is responsible for absorbing moisture. Multiple analyses are conducted to reveal the elimination of virus detection, which was determined to be 25 times greater for large aerosols and 2.5 times greater for pure particles. The four-ply surgi-cal mask consists of a three-ply face mask with an additional layer that includes an activated carbon filter or another filtering layer. The initial layer consists of polypro-pylene spun bond nonwoven material, while the second layer contains an active carbon filter fiber, or another layer designed for filtration. The third layer consists of melt-blown nonwoven fabric, while the final layer is made of polypropylene spun bond nonwoven material. In addition, they include adaptable nasal strips that pro-vide exceptional safeguarding and contentment to the wearer. Additionally, it pro-tects against both smells and organic vapors [17].

9.2.3.3 Respirators

A Filtering Facepiece Respirator (NIOSH Respirator Filter Masks)

FFP 1/2/3 or NIOSH respirators, along with other respirators, are seal-tested protec-tion devices designed to safeguard healthcare personnel, particularly those who have direct contact with patients. NIOSH respirators screening masks are respira-tory protective devices designed to contour closely to the face and provide very effective filtering of airborne particles. This device exhibits occlusion in the nasal and oral cavities and is equipped with twisted fibers containing filters [14].

With filtering facepiece (FFP) filtration is carried by using a range of intricate polypropylene microfibers and varying electrostatic rates. It is utilized for the pur-pose of removing fumes, dust particles, and medical pathogens. Furthermore, it offers the advantage of purifying the air and reducing the risk of contamination for the person wearing it [17].

Three types of FFP masks provide different levels of protection. FFP1, FFP2, and FFP3 have fold factors of 4, 10, and 20, respectively. FFP1 filters a minimum of 80% of airborne particles, while FFP2 filters a minimum of 94% of airborne parti-cles [17]. The third category of FFP3 is the most extensive precautionary measure and is the sole one advised for healthcare facilities. These devices are required to adhere to industry standards, which include rigorous testing using biological aero-sols and a maximum leakage limit of 2% [14, 18, 19].

According to the criteria of filtering particles and oil resistance performance, NIOSH respirator filters can be classified into three types: Ne, P, R.

The particle filtering efficiency is a determining factor N-type respirators can be classified into three categories: N95, N99, and N100. N95 respirators are commonly utilized in healthcare settings and are a specific type of N95 Filtering Facepiece

Respirators (FFRs), alternatively referred to as N95s [15]. The most often used type is N95, alternatively known as electret filters, which achieves a filtration efficiency of 95% for aerosols. These N90/N95 face masks are among the nine particle respirators that have been certified by NIOSH. Using a N95 mask as an illustration, the initial "N" indicates that it is not oil-resistant. A purity level of "95" indicates that the particle concentration inside the mask is 95% lower than that outside the mask when exposed to a certain number of specific test particles. The filter rate of 95% is not the standard, but rather the minimum value reached [14].

N95 does not denote a specific product name. A product may be referred to as a "N95 mask" if it satisfies the N95 standard and maintains NIOSH evaluation. A degree of safety of N95 indicates that, according to the test conditions specified in the NIOSH standard, the filter material of the mask achieves a filtration efficiency of 95% for nonoily particles (such as acid mist, dust, paint mist, microorganisms). The mask consists of four layers: inner, filter, support, and mask layer connected from outside to inside with a ventilator fan to enhance breathing [17].

Additional variations of the N95 mask include N90, valved N90, valved N95, KN90, and KN95. In the context of the N90 mask, the numerical value of 90 indicates the efficacy of the mask in removing 2.5 pm dust particles. KN90 respirators equipped with valves are particularly suitable for industries involved in nonferrous metal processing, food processing, metallurgy, construction operations, and other sources of oil and non-oil aerosol pollutants, including dust particles and smoke fog. KN90 has a particle capture rate over 90% [17, 20].

Valves in face masks, like the valved N90 and N95, have been found to allow the virus to escape from the mask. The valve functions as a "one-way valve" that primarily focuses on providing protection for the wearer, rather than actively filtering the aerosols being exhaled [14, 17, 20].

The R and P masks exhibit a certain level of resistance to oils, while the high-performance 100 model represents the smallest proportion of factors that have been evaluated under trial conditions. Three types of respirators are resistant to oil: R-type and P-type. The R-type comes in R95, R99, and R100, while the P-type comes in P95, P99, and P100. Their impressive filtering power exceeds 99% and 99.7% respectively [19]. The P100 respirator boasts an impressive filtration rate of 99.7% [17].

9.2.3.4 Face Shields
A full-length face shield is constructed with elastic headbands and a clear polycarbonate shield that extends across the face. This product effectively prevents the wearer from being exposed to coughing and other liquid droplets. It had the benefit of being lightweight and budget friendly. It is commonly utilized in a clinical setting [17]. Full-length face shields are available in various designs, all of which provide a plastic barrier to protect the face from droplets and virus particles. The faceguard coverings will provide complete coverage, extending to the chin and fitting snugly against the forehead and face-shield guard [21].

9.2.4   Importance of Wearing a Mask from a Mechanistic Perspective

Face masks and other PPE items act as a physical barrier against respiratory droplets [22]. Wearing a mask plays a crucial role in minimizing the spread of the virus. Wearing face masks was found to be the most effective preventative measure in reducing the risk of infection [23]. Wearing a face mask can significantly reduce the risk of influenza-like illness, as evidenced by a risk ratio of 0.34 and a 95% confidence interval ranging from 0.14 to 0.82 [9]. A study conducted by Eikenberry et al. indicated that the widespread adoption of masks among the public can have a substantial impact on reducing population transmission rates and death tolls [24].

Nurses should also carefully consider the potential risks and hazards associated with the consistent use of medical masks, such as:

- Potential contamination due to touching the face mask with unclean hands.
- Potential risks of not replacing medical masks when they become damp, contaminated, or damaged.
- Possible development of facial skin injuries, stinging dermatitis, or worsening acne, when used for extended periods of time.
- Masks may be uncomfortable to wear.
- The potential danger of droplet transmission and splashing to the eyes, especially when mask-wearing is not combined with proper eye protection.
- A challenge that arises when wearing them in warm and humid environments [14, 25].

9.2.5   Eye Protection

Respiratory droplets are expelled when an individual coughs, sneezes, or speaks and during some medical procedures. For instance, open suctioning of the respiratory system (where an in-line suction catheter is not employed). Research indicates that the nasal mucosa, conjunctivae, and, to a lesser extent, the oral cavity, serve as vulnerable entry points for respiratory viruses. Transmission can occur when respiratory droplets containing infectious germs are directly expelled from the patient's respiratory system and land on the vulnerable mucosal surfaces of the eye. Transmission may also occur through direct and indirect contact channels [26]. Respiratory droplets can traverse to and persist on horizontal surfaces around the patient [27].

Aggregate data supplied through the EPINet network indicates that eye exposures were frequently above 60% during the preceding 5 years. Mucocutaneous exposures reported to employee health were the biggest percentage of all nonsharp blood and/or body fluid exposures [28]. Recent data indicate that 48% of exposure accidents involved eye exposure (conjunctiva), while merely 3% of healthcare professionals utilized eye protection during these incidents [29].

The Centers for Disease Control and Prevention advocates for the utilization of personal protective equipment. During aerosol-generating procedures on patients without suspected or confirmed infections necessitating airborne precautions (e.g., M. tuberculosis, hemorrhagic fever viruses), it is advisable to utilize a face shield that completely envelops the front and sides of the face, a mask with an integrated shield, or a combination of a mask and goggles, alongside gloves and a gown [26]. Despite the absence of recommendations for Droplet Precautions concerning a particular respiratory tract pathogen, it remains essential to safeguard the eyes, nose, and mouth by employing a mask and goggles or a face shield when there is a likelihood of splashes or sprays of respiratory secretions or other bodily fluids. It is recommended that the chosen eye protection be single-use, lay-flat eye protection that incorporates a face mask with an attached shield or disposable eye protection that can be stored flat and assembled at the point of care [27].

As a best practice prevention method, instruct the nurses to incorporate eye protection when donning a mask to mitigate the risk of occupational exposure to infectious microorganisms. Furthermore, instruct the nurses to avoid intentionally touching their eyes, nose, or mouth unless hand hygiene is promptly conducted beforehand. Implementing these straightforward techniques may diminish incidences of occupational eye exposure, enhance staff safety, and lower the possibility of the ocular surface acting as a portal of entry while managing a patient with a suspected or confirmed viral respiratory illness [27].

9.2.6   Recommended Order for Application of PPE

Donning of PPE should take place outside patient rooms:

- Wear a gown that covers your body from the neck to the knees, including the arms down to the wrists. Make sure the gown also wraps around your back. Fasten the neck and waist straps, if provided.
- Choose between Mask and Respirator according to protocol from your organization. Secure straps or knots around the head and neck. Align the pliable strap with the nasal bridge to achieve an appropriate fit. Perform a thorough inspection of the respirator to ensure proper fit and functionality.
- Wear eye protection on the face to ensure sufficient protection of the face and eyes. May consist of goggles and/or a face shield.
- Make sure that the gloves are worn in a way that covers the wrist of the gown [2].

Optimal Doffing of PPE should occur outside of patient rooms:

- Take hold of the palm side of the first glove using the other gloved hand and dispose of it in the designated receptacle. Detach the second glove by inserting the fingers of the bare hand beneath the remaining glove at the wrist, then dispose of the second glove in the designated waste receptacle.

- Remove the eye protection without contamination of the outside surface on the front and hold the equipment using the strap or earpieces. Discard in a suitable recycling or garbage receptacle.
- Loosen or untie the straps or knots of the gown. To remove the gown, grasp the inner part and gently pull it away from the neck and shoulders. Invert the gown. Dispose of in a suitable receptacle.
- Avoid contact with the frontal or oral region of the mask/respirator. Detach by loosening fasteners or straps located at the rear of the head. Dispose of in the designated waste receptacle [2].

9.3   Conclusion

PPE measures guarantee the protection of patients and residents in healthcare institutions who are part of high-risk groups due to their illnesses and advanced age, from a severe infectious disease. Furthermore, this measure safeguards nurses from potentially spreading the infection. Nevertheless, the efficacy of PPE is contingent upon the availability of sufficient equipment and its proper utilization [30]. Nurses are required by law to adhere to the Occupational Health and Safety Act and its regulations about PPE [31].

References

1. Brown L. Use of personal protective equipment in nursing practice. Nurs Stand. 2019;34(5)
2. Kening MZ, Groen K. Personal protective equipment. In: StatPearls [Internet]. Treasure Island: StatPearls Publishing; 2023. PMID: 36943957.
3. Edlich R, Wind TC, Heather CL, Thacker JG. Reliability and performance of innovative surgical double-glove hole puncture indication systems. J Long-Term Eff Med Implants. 2003;13(2)
4. World Health Organization. WHO best practices for injections and related procedures toolkit. World Health Organization; 2010. Report No.: 9245599256
5. Kilinc FS. A review of isolation gowns in healthcare: fabric and gown properties. J Eng Fibers Fabrics. 2015;10(3):155892501501000313.
6. FS KB. Isolation gowns in health care settings: laboratory studies, regulations and standards, and potential barriers of gown selection and use. Am J Infect Control. 2015;44(1):104–11.
7. Kahveci Z, Kilinc-Balci FS, Yorio PL. Barrier resistance of double layer isolation gowns. Am J Infect Control. 2021;49(4):430–3.
8. Kennedy K, Vu K, Coakley N, Daley-Morris J, Forbes L, Hartzell R, et al. Safe handling of hazardous drugs. J Oncol Pharm Pract. 2023;29(2):401–12.
9. Offeddu V, Yung CF, Low MSF, Tam CC. Effectiveness of masks and respirators against respiratory infections in healthcare workers: a systematic review and meta-analysis. Clin Infect Dis. 2017;65(11):1934–42.
10. Su WC, Lee J, Xi J, Zhang K. Investigation of mask efficiency for loose-fitting masks against ultrafine particles and effect on airway deposition efficiency. Aerosol Air Qual Res. 2022 Jan;22(1):210228. https://doi.org/10.4209/aaqr.210228.
11. Andrews AS, Kiederer M, Casey ML. Understanding filtering facepiece respirators. AJN Am J Nurs. 2022;122(2):21–3.
12. Oberg T, Brosseau LM. Surgical mask filter and fit performance. Am J Infect Control. 2008;36(4):276–82.

13. Howard J, Huang A, Li Z, Tufekci Z, Zdimal V, Van Der Westhuizen H-M, et al. An evidence review of face masks against COVID-19. Proc Natl Acad Sci. 2021;118(4):e2014564118.
14. Das S, Sarkar S, Das A, Das S, Chakraborty P, Sarkar J. A comprehensive review of various categories of face masks resistant to COVID-19. Clin Epidemiol Glob Health. 2021;12:100835.
15. Shakya KM, Noyes A, Kallin R, Peltier RE. Evaluating the efficacy of cloth facemasks in reducing particulate matter exposure. J Expo Sci Environ Epidemiol. 2017;27(3):352–7.
16. Li Y-T, Linster M, Mendenhall IH, Su YC, Smith GJ. Avian influenza viruses in humans: lessons from past outbreaks. Br Med Bull. 2019;132(1):81–95.
17. Tcharkhtchi A, Abbasnezhad N, Seydani MZ, Zirak N, Farzaneh S, Shirinbayan M. An overview of filtration efficiency through the masks: mechanisms of the aerosols penetration. Bioactive Mater. 2021;6(1):106–22.
18. Gawn J, Clayton M, Makison C, Crook B. Evaluating the protection afforded by surgical masks against influenza bioaerosols: gross protection of surgical masks compared to filtering facepiece respirators. Health Saf Exec. 2008;
19. Bałazy A, Toivola M, Adhikari A, Sivasubramani SK, Reponen T, Grinshpun SA. Do N95 respirators provide 95% protection level against airborne viruses, and how adequate are surgical masks? Am J Infect Control. 2006;34(2):51–7.
20. Allison AL, Ambrose-Dempster E, Bawn M, Arredondo MC, Chau C, Chandler K, et al. The impact and effectiveness of the general public wearing masks to reduce the spread of pandemics in the UK: a multidisciplinary comparison of single-use masks versus reusable face masks. UCL Open Environ. 2021:3.
21. Lindsley WG, Noti JD, Blachere FM, Szalajda JV, Beezhold DH. Efficacy of face shields against cough aerosol droplets from a cough simulator. J Occup Environ Hyg. 2014;11(8):509–18.
22. Patel RB, Skaria SD, Mansour MM, Smaldone GC. Respiratory source control using a surgical mask: an in vitro study. J Occup Environ Hyg. 2016;13(7):569–76.
23. Seto W, Tsang D, Yung R, Ching T, Ng T, Ho M, et al. Effectiveness of precautions against droplets and contact in prevention of nosocomial transmission of severe acute respiratory syndrome (SARS). Lancet. 2003;361(9368):1519–20.
24. Eikenberry SE, Mancuso M, Iboi E, Phan T, Eikenberry K, Kuang Y, et al. To mask or not to mask: modeling the potential for face mask use by the general public to curtail the COVID-19 pandemic. Infect Dis Model. 2020;5:293–308.
25. Matusiak Ł, Szepietowska M, Krajewski PK, Białynicki-Birula R, Szepietowski JC. The use of face masks during the COVID-19 pandemic in Poland: a survey study of 2315 young adults. Dermatol Ther. 2020;33(6):e13909.
26. Siegel JD, Rhinehart E, Jackson M, Chiarello L. Guideline for isolation precautions: preventing transmission of infectious agents in healthcare settings. Last update: July 2023; 2007. p. 2023.
27. McGoldrick M. Personal protective equipment: protecting the eyes. Home Healthcare Now. 2019;37(4):234–5.
28. Mitchell AH. Improving the availability, accessibility, and use of eye protection in patient care settings. Infect Control Hosp Epidemiol. 2019;40(3):385–6.
29. Terry Grimmond F, BAgrSc G, Tr, Director G, Good L, Grimmond T. EXPO-STOP 2018–an overview of blood exposure incidence in 281 US hospitals. Streamline Your Sling Process. 2020:25.
30. Hoedl M, Eglseer D, Schoberer D, Bauer S. Factors predisposing hospitals and nursing home staff to use personal protective equipment. Collegian. 2024;31(1):20–7.
31. Dugheri S, Mucci N, Mini E, Cappelli G, Bucaletti E, Squillaci D, et al. An update on permeation of protective medical gloves by antineoplastic drugs. Sigurnost: časopis za sigurnost u radnoj i životnoj okolini. 2022;64(4):341–57.

Environmental Cleaning and Disinfection

10

Daniela Accorgi and Beatrice Meucci

10.1 Introduction

Environmental sanitization is one of the key components of standard precautions [1]. The main recommendations concern the need to establish policies and procedures for routine and targeted cleaning of environmental surfaces, based on the level of patient contact and the degree of soiling. Surfaces that could be contaminated by pathogens, including those in close proximity to patients (e.g., bed rails, nightstands) and frequently touched surfaces in the patient care environment (e.g., door handles, railings) should be cleaned and disinfected more frequently than other surfaces (e.g., horizontal surfaces in waiting rooms). Disinfectants should be used according to standards defined by regulatory bodies (e.g., CEN-European Committee for Standardization).

The purpose of environmental hygiene is to limit or eliminate microbial contamination of inanimate surfaces, so they do not become a source of pathogen transmission during patient care, to protect healthcare personnel and visitors from similar risks, and to ensure aseptic practices in a clean environment.

In the last 30 years of the past century, several publications believed that contaminated surfaces played only a negligible role in the transmission of healthcare-associated infections (HAIs) [2, 3]. Inanimate surfaces were thought to be inhospitable environments for microorganisms' survival, but a 2006 systematic review documented that common nosocomial pathogen could survive for months on surfaces in healthcare environments [4]. Subsequent reviews agreed on the microorganisms' ability to survive on any type of material present in healthcare facilities [5, 6].

Patients, staff, and visitors constantly shed microorganisms that colonize their skin and mucous membranes (microbiota), leading to environmental contamination.

D. Accorgi (✉) · B. Meucci
ANIPIO-National Scientific Society of Nurse Infectious Risk Specialists, Bologna, Italy

© The Author(s), under exclusive license to Springer Nature Switzerland AG 2025
B. Oomen, S. Gastaldi (eds.), *Principles of Nursing Infection Prevention Control*,
Principles of Specialty Nursing, https://doi.org/10.1007/978-3-031-84469-0_10

The surface area of human skin covers about 1.8 m^2. Together with hair follicles, sebaceous glands, and other appendages, human skin provides a habitat for more than 10^{10} microbes, with 1 million microbes present per cm^2. Most people release 30,000–60,000 dead skin cells every minute, equivalent to over 500 million per day. These dead skin cells are continuously dispersed as small dust particles, settling in any environment where people reside. About 10% of dead skin cells contain bacteria, ranging from 5 to 12 bacteria per cell [7].

The total surface area of mucous membranes in a human is about 400 m^2 and hosts varying numbers of microorganisms depending on the organ system. For example, the stomach contains $\sim$10^1–10^3 colony-forming units (CFU)/mL. The duodenum has concentrations of around 10^1–10^3 CFU/mL, while the jejunum has concentrations of 10^4–10^7 CFU/mL. The colon presents the highest concentration, with 10^9–10^{12} CFU/mL [8].

Microorganisms colonizing the mucous membranes are dispersed into the environment through body fluids during physiological or pathological actions, such as sneezing, coughing, defecating, urinating, or vomiting. Therefore, the environment is continually contaminated by human microorganisms.

Additionally, numerous invasive procedures (e.g., surgeries, insertion and management of medical devices) increase the potential for body fluids to come into contact with the environment, leading to contamination with microorganisms if contaminated instruments and waste materials are not properly managed. Infected individuals (e.g., Clostridioides difficile infection) can further disperse pathogenic microorganisms into the environment through infectious symptoms (e.g., diarrhea). When the population residing in healthcare environments has been or is being treated with antibiotics, the microorganisms contaminating the environment may exhibit antibiotic resistance.

Healthcare facilities' indoor environments thus tend to become contaminated with many microorganisms, often with important resistance profiles. These facilities also host individuals more susceptible to infection due to their medical conditions and the diagnostic and treatment interventions they undergo. Inanimate surfaces, such as equipment, medical devices, and furniture around patients, are more prone to contamination than other areas of the facility, both because of microbiota dispersion and because these surfaces are frequently "touched" by hands (with or without gloves) of healthcare personnel, patients, and visitors.

If individuals adhered optimally to hand hygiene guidelines, the risk of indirect contact transmission from inanimate surfaces would be minimal. However, the literature shows that healthcare worker adherence to the five moments of hand hygiene averages around 40% [9]. This highlights that while efforts to improve hand hygiene are important, we must also consider the environmental hygiene interventions implemented in our facilities to mitigate transmission risks. Some authors suggest that a multimodal environmental cleaning strategy is needed to better respond to these risks [10].

Some authors emphasize that the inanimate environment is not only contaminated but can also play a role in microorganism transmission. Otter et al. [11] were among the first to highlight that the transmission route of Clostridioides difficile, multidrug-resistant microorganisms such as Methicillin-Resistant *Staphylococcus aureus* (MRSA) and Vancomycin-resistant Enterococcus (VRE), some Gram-negative bacteria, and Norovirus from colonized/infected patients to susceptible individuals is linked to contamination of surfaces and healthcare equipment [11]. Subsequent publications [12–18] and two meta-analyses [19, 20] confirmed this correlation. According to an initial review by Carling [21], patients occupying rooms previously occupied by patients colonized or infected with vancomycin-resistant Enterococcus, MRSA, *C. difficile*, or *Acinetobacter baumannii* had a 73% higher risk of acquiring a pathogenic microorganism compared to patients who had not [21].

Attention shifted to the quality of environmental cleaning services, which in the early 1990s were considered primarily an aesthetic necessity, as Dancer recalled [22]. Carling's 2010 [21] review also noted that only 40% of near-patient surfaces were cleaned correctly, and an 82% improvement in cleaning was associated with a 68% reduction in environmental contamination of "high-risk equipment" [21]. Donskey's systematic review found that environmental disinfection is an effective risk control strategy for C. difficile, MRSA, VRE, and Norovirus, though it remains unclear when environmental disinfection should occur [23].

One of the most recent studies on this topic comes from Australia. The REACH (Researching Effective Approaches to Cleaning in Hospitals) study clearly demonstrated the crucial role of thorough environmental cleaning in preventing HAIs. Implementing a multimodal cleaning package—comprising technical training, product use, audits, and communication—not only improved the performance, knowledge, and attitude of environmental services staff but also reduced the incidence of clinically significant hospital pathogens [24].

As noted by Assadian et al. [2], there are no universally accepted guidelines or recommendations for surface cleaning and disinfection. As such, expert guidance can be helpful in daily practice to define standard principles for cleaning and disinfection, technical-operational methods, operator training, and evaluation systems.

We will refer to six key documents: the recommendations of the Provincial Infectious Diseases Advisory Committee (PIDAC) of Ontario, Canada [25], the Commission for Hospital Hygiene and Infection Prevention (KRINKO) [26], and the Robert Koch Institute's German recommendations, the UK National Health Service [27], the Australian Commission on Safety and Quality in Health Care [28], the U.S. Centers for Disease Control and Prevention [29], and the Italian National Association of Medical Directors along with other Italian scientific societies [30].

The key elements we will describe are the following:

1. Risk assessment and classification criteria.
2. Objectives to achieve through sanitization.
3. Principles of technical-operational methodology.
4. Organization of the external provider's sanitization service.
5. Criteria for selecting equipment, materials, and products.
6. Cleaning frequency.
7. Training and education of staff.

8. Evaluation and control measures.
9. Responsibilities.

10.2   Risk Assessment and Surface/Area Classification Criteria

As with other infection risk prevention and control interventions, it is necessary to establish criteria to identify actions to mitigate or eliminate risk.

Assadian et al. [2] propose a risk assessment model based on three essential factors:

(a) Patient-related risk (e.g., patient with infection or colonization).
(b) Surface-related risk (e.g., likelihood of contamination with pathogenic micro-organisms, potential exposure or indirect transmission, frequency of hand contact).
(c) Pathogen-related risk (e.g., antibiotic resistance, mode of transmission).

These three factors are interdependent, and all must be considered when assessing the risk for specific areas (e.g., wards, services) and surfaces (e.g., equipment, medical devices).

At least three risk levels for areas/surfaces are defined: high, medium, and low risk. In some documents, up to six levels are identified.

Moderate to high-risk areas include patient rooms with bathrooms, wards hosting immunosuppressed patients or those in intensive care, and bone marrow transplant units. Operating rooms and clean rooms are considered high-risk areas. It is important to note that "high-risk rooms" can also be found in moderate-risk areas. For example, a patient room previously occupied by a patient with multidrug-resistant microorganisms or C. difficile may pose a higher infection/colonization risk to newly admitted patients.

Low-risk areas are those where no patient care activities take place, such as administrative offices and hallways.

In surface risk assessment, it is necessary to distinguish between high-contact and low-contact surfaces. High-contact surfaces can further be classified as critical, semi-critical, and noncritical (based on Spaulding's criteria) [31].

– Low-contact surfaces: These are not handled by the patient or healthcare staff and are unlikely to come into contact with skin (e.g., floors, walls, or environmental surfaces outside the point of care).
– High-contact surfaces, on the other hand, are usually close to the patient, frequently touched by the patient or healthcare staff, and come into contact with the skin. Due to the increased contact, they pose a particularly high risk of pathogen transmission. Examples of high-contact surfaces in the point of care include bed rails, door handles, nightstands, biomedical equipment, and patient-exclusive medical devices. Outside the point of care, high-contact surfaces to be

considered include elevator buttons and handrails. The transmission risk from high-contact surfaces also depends on their use in relation to care or assistance procedures.

Spaulding defines noncritical surfaces as those that only come into contact with intact skin, presenting a low infection risk. Semi-critical surfaces are those that come into contact with intact mucous membranes and non-intact skin. Finally, critical surfaces come into direct contact with blood or mucous membranes or with sterile medical devices (e.g., needles, vascular access devices).

Surface risk classification should include surfaces or elements (equipment, furniture, and devices) that will be cleaned by external providers and those that will be handled by internal staff. The goal is to ensure microbial load reduction to guarantee safe care.

10.3   Objectives to Achieve Through Sanitization

All areas and surfaces must be cleaned and washed to remove organic and inorganic substances deposited on surfaces. Disinfection represents a secondary measure, to be applied after cleaning and washing when the presence of microorganisms on surfaces does not guarantee care safety, and a disinfectant is applied to clean surfaces. For critical surfaces, safety is ensured through sterilization (see Table 10.1— Definition of Sanitization Objectives).

The main goal of sanitization is dirt removal. Dirt has certain characteristics that must be understood to select the most appropriate equipment, materials, and products.

Dirt refers to the presence of organic or inorganic substances that, when deposited or adhered to an object's surface, degrade its appearance and compromise hygiene, leading to progressive deterioration over time. A criterion for classifying

Table 10.1 Definition of sanitization objectives

Definition of sanitization and objectives	
Cleaning	Activities involving procedures and operations to remove and eliminate waste, dust, and dirt of any kind, whether adhered or not, from confined and non-confined surface environments.
Washing	Operation aimed at eliminating any traces of dirt (adhered dirt) from substrates to make them visually clean through chemical action, adequate mechanical action, and a specific time of action, without altering their physical characteristics.
Disinfection	A procedure intended to eliminate or destroy pathogenic microorganisms but not necessarily all microbial forms (e.g., bacterial endospores) on inanimate objects through the application of appropriate physical or chemical agents (e.g., heat, disinfectants).
Sterilization	The process of killing all microorganisms through physical or chemical means. Sterilization is used only for critical items, that is, objects or instruments that enter or penetrate sterile tissues, cavities, or the bloodstream.

Table designed by the author'

Table 10.2 Types of dirt

Types of dirt	
Loose dirt	Particles or materials that settle on surfaces without adhering to them. It can be divided into coarse and fine dirt. Removing it does not require chemical or physical intervention, just simple mechanical action with appropriate equipment:
Coarse	Composed of residues such as stones, sand, cigarette butts, paper, work residues, textile residues.
Fine	Dust of various types and different origins that settle on surfaces.
Adhered dirt	Composed of organic and inorganic substances that cling to the surface. Removing it requires the use of chemicals and/or physical means for mechanical dirt removal.
Crusted dirt	Dirt that has penetrated the porous part of surfaces and consists of hard water or carbon residues often mixed with dust and grease. This type of dirt is difficult to remove and requires specific products.

Table designed by the author

dirt is its ability to adhere to surfaces, which allows it to be categorized as shown in Table 10.2—Types of Dirt.

Dust particles range in size from 0.25 to 500 microns. To the naked eye, we can perceive particles as small as 5 microns, which is why dust is often present even where we don't notice it. Dead skin cells constitute a large percentage of dust and are released in large quantities by patients, staff, and visitors. These particles settle on all surfaces and can act as potential vectors for microorganism transport. Once settled, dust should not be recirculated, as air movement can recontaminate surfaces or be inhaled by people [7].

Regarding disinfection, one emerging challenge is the formation of biofilms by microorganisms. A biofilm is a matrix composed of extracellular polymeric substances containing polysaccharides, proteins, lipids, enzymes, extracellular DNA, and water. This matrix encapsulates the microbial community that formed it, providing protection and nutrients. This protective layer prevents disinfectants and antibiotics from effectively destroying microorganisms. It is estimated that 65–80% of all bacterial and chronic infections derive from biofilms. Biofilms can form on both wet and dry environmental surfaces, as first described in 2012. The best strategy to prevent biofilm formation is still under investigation, but effective mechanical action on surfaces, especially dry biofilms, is considered a good preventive measure [32, 33].

10.4 Principles of the Technical-Operational Methodology (Products and Processes)

The type of equipment and products used is selected based on the classification of the area/surface, but the principles that govern the technical-operational methodology are the same:

A. Proceed from the cleanest point to the dirtiest. This helps prevent the spread of dirt and microorganisms.

B. Proceed from top to bottom. This avoids dirt and microorganisms from "falling" or contaminating already cleaned areas.

C. Work methodically and systematically. This ensures that no areas are missed during sanitization.

1. Dusting techniques must not spread dust, so it is necessary to use damp or antistatic cloths.

2. Dusting, cleaning, and disinfection of large, flat surfaces should be done using "S"-shaped movements, starting from the farthest point, overlapping slightly without returning to the area to avoid recontamination.

3. Frequently touched points (high-touch surfaces), such as door handles, call buttons, light switches, bed rails, and nightstands, should be cleaned more frequently than other surfaces.

4. A color-coding system should be used for all equipment and materials (e.g., buckets and reusable cloths) according to their primary use to prevent cross-contamination.

5. Floors should be cleaned last.

10.5 Organization—External Provider's Sanitization Service

The external provider must have a service area for the reconditioning of reusable equipment and materials, material storage, and administrative activities (e.g., staff shift management).

The reconditioning area is where contaminated/dirty equipment must be treated to be reused. Therefore, it is necessary to establish clear identification of clean/dirty paths and areas of low and high contamination. There should be a reusable cloth washing system subject to biocontamination monitoring and control, as required by the EN 14065 standard [34], and an automatic dilution system for detergents and disinfectants.

10.6 Criteria for Selecting Equipment, Materials, and Products

The selection and appropriate use of supplies and equipment are essential for effective cleaning programs. Equipment must be ergonomic, easy to disassemble and reassemble to allow efficient reconditioning. Prefer items that have a lower environmental impact, in line with environmental protection policies. The number of different products should be minimized, and those with lower toxicity levels for staff should be prioritized.

• Equipped Cart: Equipment, materials, and products must be transported from the external provider's service area to the usage area and vice versa. For this, a modular equipped cart is recommended. It must allow the transport of all items necessary for service provision and the collection of waste and contaminated cloths.

The cart must be organized to separate clean materials and products from dirty ones.

- Floor Cleaning Systems: The system consists of an adjustable telescopic handle and a swivel frame for placing floor cloths. The cloth can be dampened with the cleaning solution using a double-bucket system or, to reduce cross-contamination and water consumption, a container where the cloths are pre-soaked before starting activities.
- Surface Cleaning Equipment: United Kingdom's National Health Service (NHS) in 2021 [35], defined a Color-coded buckets system for high-risk surfaces are preferable, such as:
  - Red: Bathrooms, toilets, showers, sinks, and bathroom floors.
  - Blue: General areas, wards, departments, offices, and public areas.
  - Green: Ward kitchens and catering services for patients in the ward areas.
  - Yellow: Isolation areas.

In selecting the quality of floor and surface cloths, it is important to facilitate the removal of loose dirt and to remove adhered dirt through mechanical action. Microfiber's physical characteristics represent an optimal solution compared to cotton and disposable nonwoven fabrics (TNT), for example. Microfiber is a technical fiber with a denier value equal to or less than 1 Dtex (decitex) (EN ISO 10714) [36]. This technical measurement unit refers to the ratio between the fiber's length and density. The Dtex system indicates how many meters of a particular fiber are contained in 1 g of weight: 1 Dtex equals 10,000 m. The most common type of microfiber consists of a variable component of polyamide and polyester fibers combined into a single thread. During the production process, these thin threads are split, producing multi-filament fibers that, when viewed cross-sectionally under a microscope, resemble a "star." This shape creates millions of "pockets" where dirt and microorganisms are collected, which are released only after machine washing, provided the correct temperature and detergents are used to clean and maintain the star-shaped form.

- Detergents: These are chemical products in an aqueous solution for the removal of adhered dirt. One of the main components is surfactants. A surfactant consists of a hydrophilic part that binds to water and a hydrophobic part that tends to bind to the fatty part of the dirt, facilitating solubilization. Fatty dirt dissolves in the lipophilic tails, and the particles are dispersed in water via the hydrophilic part. Depending on the type of dirt and surface, different types of surfactants are used with the same goal of "detaching" the adhered dirt without damaging the surfaces. Currently, no standardized tests exist to evaluate the reduction of microbial load after cleaning.
- Disinfectants: Dirt removal reduces the microbial load on areas/surfaces, making them safe for patients, staff, and visitors, and minimizing people's exposure to chemical substances. For some areas/surfaces and patient types, it may be useful to combine cleaning with disinfection. This applies to areas like operating rooms, intensive care units, and wards hosting patients with severe immunosuppression,

neutropenia, etc. Disinfection always complements cleaning operations and does not replace them unless it involves a combined detergent-disinfectant product. For disinfectants, standardized tests exist to evaluate microbial load. These tests are required by manufacturers for market authorization in relation to their intended use. The reference standard that summarizes all tests related to intended use is EN 14885 [37], and other standards for demonstrating biocide efficacy are indicated in the ECHA document [38]. Disinfection should achieve a reduction of vegetative bacteria on the surface by ≥ 5 log10. For yeasts, molds, mycobacteria, *C. difficile* spores, and viruses, the requirement is set at ≥ 4 log10. EN 14885 [37] lists the mandatory tests for each specific use case and optional tests, as well as the type of microorganisms for evaluating outcomes. The main European regulation governing disinfectant use is the Biocidal Products Regulation and the Medical Devices Regulation [39].

To select the most appropriate disinfectant product, we must distinguish between surfaces that are not certified as medical devices (and thus do not bear the CE mark) and those that are registered as medical devices (which bear the CE mark). For non-CE marked surfaces, biocides registered as type 2 products should generally be used, following the Biocidal Products Regulation [39].

Disinfectants used on CE-marked equipment and medical devices are considered "accessories" of the device itself, and for their authorization, the same regulations apply. Users must employ disinfectants authorized as Medical Devices (MD). A disinfectant may be declared both as an MD and as a biocide (indicating dual-use products). This means that different requirement profiles may exist. Disinfectants for surfaces declared for processing MDs must be approved as MDs and meet the requirements of the Medical Devices Regulation (MDR). The MD's compliance with essential safety and performance requirements is confirmed by the manufacturer with the CE mark and a declaration of conformity. Disinfectants for MDs not only require an efficacy declaration but also a compatibility declaration with the MD, such as storage stability after opening. Disinfectants should be used according to technical specifications and in compliance with the Safety Data Sheet information concerning risks to people and the environment [40].

Most detergents and disinfectants used for cleaning are aqueous solutions and are not ready-to-use. Therefore, they must be diluted just before use in dedicated areas and at the correct concentration, which makes having automatic dilution systems beneficial. These systems require maintenance and verification of the dosing system's performance. Standardized containers (for measuring solutions) and easy-to-use visual aids (e.g., posters) should be used for solution preparation.

In recent years the disinfectant products are increasingly being offered not just as solutions containing one or more active ingredients but also as "disinfection systems," meaning products that combine the chemical action of the active ingredient and mechanical application for surface treatment. Tests have been defined to evaluate the efficacy of these systems. Ready-to-use disinfectant wipes are tested for efficacy, such as the EN 16615: 2015 standard, which only evaluates bactericidal and yeasticidal action [41]. Automated "no-touch" disinfection systems containing active ingredients are tested according to specific standards [42].

10.7   Cleaning Frequency

The main cleaning frequencies are categorized as follows: regular cleaning in patient wards, cleaning upon discharge/transfer, periodic cleaning, and extraordinary cleaning.

- Regular cleaning in patient wards: This cleaning is performed according to a schedule, which can be daily for areas where patients are always present or where care activities are conducted. It focuses on areas where the patient resides, including the floor, surfaces near the patient, and dedicated bathrooms. To facilitate this type of cleaning, internal staff must ensure that external service operators can access the items to be cleaned, such as by minimizing clutter on nightstands or floors.
- Cleaning upon discharge/transfer: After a patient is discharged, deep cleaning can be performed on surfaces occupied by the patient to remove organic material and significantly reduce or eliminate microbial contamination, ensuring that there is no transfer of microorganisms to the next patient. Disposable patient care items should be discarded, and equipment and devices used during the patient's care should be removed for reprocessing.
- Scheduled or periodic cleaning: Scheduled cleaning takes place alongside regular or terminal cleaning and aims to reduce dust and dirt on low-contact objects or surfaces. Perform scheduled cleaning on objects or surfaces that are not typically at risk of dirt, using neutral detergents and water. However, if these surfaces are visibly soiled with blood or body fluids, they should be cleaned and disinfected as soon as possible. The frequency of scheduled cleaning can vary: weekly, monthly, semi-annual, or annual.
- Extraordinary cleaning: This refers to cleaning or disinfection after special events, such as renovations, flooding, or outbreaks of microorganisms, where there is suspicion of an environmental reservoir. These cleanings must be coordinated with the Infection Prevention and Control Team, the external provider, and facility managers.

10.8   Training and Education of Personnel

Proper training and education of personnel involved in cleaning and disinfection are essential to ensure the effectiveness of infection prevention and control measures. Both external provider staff and internal healthcare personnel must have a clear understanding of their roles and responsibilities in maintaining hygiene standards. Since cleaning tasks are often performed manually, staff must be adequately trained to follow procedures correctly and use cleaning products and equipment safely and effectively. It is also important to regularly evaluate the training programs to ensure continuous adherence to the required standards. Below are the key considerations for the training and education of both external and internal staff:

- External provider cleaning staff: Cleaning staff are the frontline in infection prevention and control, so it is crucial to focus on their education and training, as most cleaning procedures are performed manually by operators. A training program must be scheduled for every new hire or whenever new equipment, or products are introduced. The training must consider the adult population, including any potential language or cultural barriers. Training and learning assessments should be documented.
- Internal personnel: Internal staff must be aware of the elements that need to be cleaned and/or disinfected within the healthcare facility. Internal procedures must be defined to outline the responsibilities of interventions and how they should be implemented. Product technical sheets and safety data sheets must be made available. Training courses with learning assessments must be provided.

10.9 Measures for Evaluation and Control

Regularly evaluating the cleaning process allows verification of adherence to established standards and the scheduling of improvement interventions, if necessary. Various evaluation and control methods are proposed, each with its advantages and disadvantages, as they examine different aspects of the cleaning process. Due to the unique characteristics of each control system, it is reasonable to use them in combination, particularly when the service is outsourced to an external provider [43, 44]. The following is an explanation of the key methods mentioned:

(a) Audit through visual inspection: Visual inspection audits are the most cost-effective method to evaluate cleanliness and are the quickest way to identify severe deficiencies in an area. However, this method is subjective and does not detect bacterial load. It identifies the presence of visible dirt, dust, waste, stains, and moisture.
(b) Direct observation during interventions: Using a checklist, operators' adherence to defined procedures is observed. Observation can be carried out both during the cleaning of healthcare environments and in the reconditioning and preparation area for equipment.
(c) User surveys: Satisfaction surveys assess patient/resident/family satisfaction with the cleanliness of an environment. These surveys are often part of a broader survey on environmental satisfaction and include questions related to cleanliness. Results can be aggregated and shared with staff and stakeholders.
(d) ATP testing: This involves using a swab to detect biological residue on surfaces. The system measures the presence of ATP (adenosine triphosphate), an energy molecule present in all animals, plant, bacterial cells, yeasts, and molds. The analysis system uses the chemiluminescence capability of the

luciferin-luciferase reagent, which emits light when it comes into contact with ATP; the intensity of the emitted light is directly proportional to the amount of ATP present. The swabs are placed in a detection device that measures the light emission (measured in relative light units or RLU).

(e) Microbiological sampling using contact plates: This is done by applying contact Petri dishes (with the surface of the medium suitable for adhesion with the surface to be monitored), filled with an appropriate culture medium, by applying slight pressure on the surface. They can be used on flat surfaces.

(f) Microbiological sampling using swabs: Swabs, moistened with a neutralizing solution, are swiped over a 100 cm^2 surface. To ensure proper sampling, it is important to use a crosshatch motion to cover the entire surface of interest.

(g) Fluorescent markers: This method uses an invisible transparent gel applied to critical points in the environment to be sanitized. It dries on surfaces and resists dry abrasion but can be easily removed with slight abrasion after wetting. The gel is visible only under ultraviolet (UV) light, so the completeness of the cleaning can be determined by using UV light on the areas where the gel was applied before cleaning.

10.10 Responsibility

Cleaning and disinfection of the environment, understood as a measure to prevent infection risk, are carried out by both external providers and internal staff. Therefore, it is necessary to clarify not only the working methods but also who holds responsibility for process evaluation and improvement measures. The WHO Guidelines on Core Components of Infection Prevention and Control Programs at the National and Acute Healthcare Facility Level should guide the Infection Prevention and Control Team in the interventions for which they are responsible [45].

10.11 Conclusions

Although environmental sanitization is one of the key components of standard precautions, there are critical factors that can compromise the effectiveness of this intervention. Evaluation of outsourcing these activities based on risk assessment has shown that adherence to defined measures rarely reaches the standards, increasing the risk that the environment becomes a source of microorganism transmission. Careful training and education of external provider personnel have improved operator adherence to defined standards and reduced environmental contamination of equipment, especially at the point of care. Certain elements, particularly high-touch surfaces, as they are more frequently contaminated, require careful risk assessment and the inclusion of sanitization and disinfection interventions by internal staff. Improving staff adherence to the five moments of hand hygiene reduces the risk of transmission related to high-touch surfaces. The formation of biofilm poses a challenge to the effectiveness of disinfectants, and it is essential to prevent biofilm formation, although the most effective measures, particularly for dry biofilms, are still to be clearly defined.

References

1. Siegel JD, Rhinehart E, Jackson M, Chiarello L. & health care infection control practices advisory committee. Guideline for isolation precautions: preventing transmission of infectious agents in health care settings. Am J Infect Control. 2007;35(10 Suppl 2):S65–S164. https://doi.org/10.1016/j.ajic.2007.10.007.
2. Assadian O, Harbarth S, Vos M, Knobloch JK, Asensio A, Widmer AF. Practical recommendations for routine cleaning and disinfection procedures in healthcare institutions: a narrative review. J Hosp Infect. 2021;113:104–14. https://doi.org/10.1016/j.jhin.2021.03.010.
3. Dancer SJ. Hospital cleaning: past, present, and future. Antimicrob Resist Infect Control. 2023;12(1):80. https://doi.org/10.1186/s13756-023-01275-3.
4. Porter L, Sultan O, Mitchell BG, Jenney A, Kiernan M, Brewster DJ, Russo PL. How long do nosocomial pathogens persist on inanimate surfaces? A scoping review. J Hosp Infect. 2024;147:25–31. https://doi.org/10.1016/j.jhin.2024.01.023.
5. Wißmann JE, Kirchhoff L, Brüggemann Y, Todt D, Steinmann J, Steinmann E. Persistence of pathogens on inanimate surfaces: a narrative review. Microorganisms. 2021;9(2):343. https://doi.org/10.3390/microorganisms9020343.
6. Kramer A, Schwebke I, Kampf G. How long do nosocomial pathogens persist on inanimate surfaces? A systematic review. BMC Infect Dis. 2006;6:130. https://doi.org/10.1186/1471-2334-6-130.
7. Andersen BM. Cleaning of rooms in wards. In: Prevention and control of infections in hospitals. Cham: Springer; 2019. https://doi.org/10.1007/978-3-319-99921-0_65.
8. Martinez-Guryn K, Leone V, Chang EB. Regional diversity of the gastrointestinal microbiome. Cell Host Microbe. 2019;26(3):314–24. https://doi.org/10.1016/j.chom.2019.08.011.
9. World Health Organization. WHO guidelines on hand hygiene in health care: first global patient safety challenge clean care is safer care. World Health Organization; 2009.
10. Browne K, Mitchell BG. Multimodal environmental cleaning strategies to prevent healthcare-associated infections. Antimicrob Resist Infect Control. 2023;12(1):83. https://doi.org/10.1186/s13756-023-01274-4.
11. Otter JA, Yezli S, French GL. The role played by contaminated surfaces in the transmission of nosocomial pathogens. Infect Control Hosp Epidemiol. 2011;32(7):687–99. https://doi.org/10.1086/660363.
12. Otter JA, Yezli S, Salkeld JA, French GL. Evidence that contaminated surfaces contribute to the transmission of hospital pathogens and an overview of strategies to address contaminated surfaces in hospital settings. Am J Infect Control. 2013;41(Suppl 5):S6–S11. https://doi.org/10.1016/j.ajic.2012.12.004.
13. Weber DJ, Anderson D, Rutala WA. The role of the surface environment in healthcare-associated infections. Curr Opin Infect Dis. 2013;26(4):338–44. https://doi.org/10.1097/QCO.0b013e3283630f04.
14. Nseir S, Blazejewski C, Lubret R, Wallet F, Courcol R, Durocher A. Risk of acquiring multidrug-resistant gram-negative bacilli from prior room occupants in the intensive care unit. Clin Microbiol Infect. 2011;17(8):1201–8. https://doi.org/10.1111/j.1469-0691.2010.03420.x.
15. Datta R, Platt R, Yokoe DS, Huang SS. Environmental cleaning intervention and risk of acquiring multidrug-resistant organisms from prior room occupants. Arch Intern Med. 2011;171(6):491–4. https://doi.org/10.1001/archinternmed.2011.64.
16. Cohen B, Cohen CC, Løyland B, Larson EL. Transmission of health care-associated infections from roommates and prior room occupants: a systematic review. Clin Epidemiol. 2017;9:297–310. https://doi.org/10.2147/CLEP.S124382.

17. Cohen B, Liu J, Cohen AR, Larson E. Association between healthcare-associated infection and exposure to hospital roommates and previous bed occupants with the same organism. Infect Control Hosp Epidemiol. 2018;39(5):541–6. https://doi.org/10.1017/ice.2018.22.
18. Drees M, Snydman DR, Schmid CH, Barefoot L, Hansjosten K, Vue PM, Cronin M, Nasraway SA, Golan Y. Prior environmental contamination increases the risk of acquisition of vancomycin-resistant enterococci. Clin Infect Dis. 2008;46(5):678–85. https://doi.org/10.1086/527394.
19. Mitchell BG, Dancer SJ, Anderson M, Dehn E. Risk of organism acquisition from prior room occupants: a systematic review and meta-analysis. J Hosp Infect. 2015;91(3):211–7. https://doi.org/10.1016/j.jhin.2015.08.005.
20. Wu YL, Yang XY, Ding XX, Li RJ, Pan MS, Zhao X, Hu XQ, Zhang JJ, Yang LQ. Exposure to infected/colonized roommates and prior room occupants increases the risks of healthcare-associated infections with the same organism. J Hosp Infect. 2019;101(2):231–9. https://doi.org/10.1016/j.jhin.2018.10.014.
21. Carling PC, Bartley JM. Evaluating hygienic cleaning in health care settings: what you do not know can harm your patients. Am J Infect Control. 2010;38(5 Suppl 1):S50. https://doi.org/10.1016/j.ajic.2010.03.004.
22. Dancer SJ. Controlling hospital-acquired infection: focus on the role of the environment and new technologies for decontamination. Clin Microbiol Rev. 2014;27(4):665–90. https://doi.org/10.1128/CMR.00020-14.
23. Donskey CJ. Does improving surface cleaning and disinfection reduce health care-associated infections? Am J Infect Control. 2013;41(Suppl 5):S19. https://doi.org/10.1016/j.ajic.2012.12.010.
24. Hall L, White NM, Allen M, Farrington A, Mitchell BG, Page K, Halton K, Riley TV, Gericke CA, Graves N, Gardner A. Effectiveness of a structured, framework-based approach to implementation: the researching effective approaches to cleaning in hospitals (REACH) trial. Antimicrob Resist Infect Control. 2020;9(1):35. https://doi.org/10.1186/s13756-020-0694-0.
25. Provincial Infectious Diseases Advisory Committee (PIDAC). Best practices for environmental cleaning for prevention and control of infections in all health care settings. Ontario: 3 Public Health Ontario; 2018. https://www.publichealthontario.ca/-/media/documents/B/2018/bp-environmental-cleaning.pdf
26. Commission for Hospital Hygiene and Infection Prevention (KRINKO). Hygiene requirements for cleaning and disinfection of surfaces: recommendation of the Commission for Hospital Hygiene and Infection Prevention (KRINKO) at the Robert Koch Institute. GMS Hyg Infect Control. 2024:19. https://doi.org/10.3205/dgkh000468.
27. NHS. National Standards of healthcare cleanliness 2021. England NHS; 2021. https://www.england.nhs.uk/estates/national-standards-of-healthcare-cleanliness-2021/
28. ANMDO. Sanitization of healthcare environment: technical standards, monitoring and management of clinical risk. Issuu. 2023; https://issuu.com/edicomsrl/docs/sanificazione_interno?fr=sZDQxNDE2MzQyMzQ
29. Australian Commission on Safety and Quality in Health Care. Environmental cleaning and infection prevention and control, environmental cleaning and infection prevention and control resources. Saf Qual. 2023; https://www.safetyandquality.gov.au/our-work/infection-prevention-and-control/environmental-cleaning-and-infection-prevention-and-control-resources
30. CDC Atlanta. Environmental cleaning procedures. CDC; 2024. https://www.cdc.gov/healthcare-associated-infections/hcp/cleaning-global/procedures.html
31. Rowan NJ, Kremer T, McDonnell G. A review of Spaulding's classification system for effective cleaning, disinfection and sterilization of reusable medical devices: viewed through a modern-day lens that will inform and enable future sustainability. Sci Total Environ. 2023;878:162976. https://doi.org/10.1016/j.scitotenv.2023.162976.
32. Maillard JY, Centeleghe I. How biofilm changes our understanding of cleaning and disinfection. Antimicrob Resist Infect Control. 2023;12(1):95. https://doi.org/10.1186/s13756-023-01290-4.

33. Jamal M, Ahmad W, Andleeb S, Jalil F, Imran M, Nawaz MA, Hussain T, Ali M, Rafiq M, Kamil MA. Bacterial biofilm and associated infections. J Chinese Med Assoc: JCMA. 2018;81(1):7–11. https://doi.org/10.1016/j.jcma.2017.07.012.

34. EN 14065. Textiles. Laundry processed textiles. Biocontamination control system; 2002.

35. United Kingdom's National Health System, National Standards of healthcare cleanliness 2021: Appendices, April 2022, https://www.england.nhs.uk/wp-content/uploads/2021/04/B0271-national-standards-of-healthcare-cleanliness-2021-appendicies-april-2021.pdf

36. EN ISO 10714:2024, Steel and iron—Determination of phosphorus content—Phosphovanadomolybdate spectrophotometric method (ISO 10714:2024), 2024.

37. EN 14885: 2022. Chemical disinfectants and antiseptics. Application of European Standard for chemical disinfectants and antiseptics.

38. ECHA. Guidance Regulation on the Volume II: Efficacy Parts B+C: Assessment and Evaluation Version 6.0, August 2023.

39. Regulation (EU) No 528/2012 of the European Parliament and of the Council of 22 May 2012 concerning the making available on the market and use of biocidal products. OJ L 167, 27.6.2012. pp. 1–123.

40. Regulation (EU) No 2017/745 of the European Parliament and of the Council of 5 April 2017 on medical devices, amending Directive 2001/83/EC, Regulation (EC) No 178/2002 and Regulation (EC) No 1223/2009 and repealing Council Directives 90/385/EEC and 93/42/EEC. *OJ L 117*, 5.5.2017, p. 1–175.

41. EN—EN 16615. Chemical disinfectants and antiseptics—Quantitative test method for the evaluation of bactericidal and yeasticidal activity on non-porous surfaces with mechanical action employing wipes in the medical area (4- field test)—Test method and requirements (phase 2, step 2).

42. EN 17272: 2020. Determining the biocidal activity of Automated Airborne Room Disinfection Process.

43. Brett GM, Wilson F, Dancer SJ, McGregor A. Methods to evaluate environmental cleanliness in healthcare facilities. Healthcare Infect. 2013;18(1):23–30.

44. Carling P. Methods for assessing the adequacy of practice and improving room disinfection. Am J Infect Control. 2013;41(Suppl 5):S25. https://doi.org/10.1016/j.ajic.2013.01.003.

45. Guidelines on core components of infection prevention and control Programmes at the National and Acute Health Care Facility Level. World Health Organization; 2016.

Historical Context and Improving Hand Hygiene Compliance Through Positive Deviance Approach

11

Noel Abela

11.1 Introduction

Ignaz Semmelweis (1818—1865) and Florence Nightingale (1820—1910) were both pioneers in promoting handwashing as preventative measures to stop the transmission of infections. This theory has been used across all healthcare institutions, and during the SARS-CoV-2 pandemic, hand hygiene was promoted as one of the ways to stop transmission.

11.2 Ignaz Semmelweis—The Father of Hand Hygiene

Ignaz Semmelweis (1818—1865) may not have a well-known name, but today's healthcare settings benefit greatly from his work. He was born in Buda (now Budapest) in Hungary and obtained his medical degree at the University of Vienna in 1844. He later worked at the Vienna General Hospital, where he made groundbreaking observations regarding the transmission of puerperal fever.

When he started working as an assistant to a professor in the maternity ward, the First Department in 1846, he was confronted with a dire situation; 13–18% of women delivered by physicians and medical students died as a result of childbed fever (puerperal fever). In the second department, there were no doctors or students and women were assisted during delivery by midwives and trainee-midwives', and the mortality rate was approximately 2% [1].

Semmelwies managed to solve this mystery when he learned that his colleague and friend Jakob Kolletschka, who supervised medical students in the mortuary room, sustained a cut injury and eventually died from puerperal fever. Semmelweis

N. Abela (✉)
Faculty of Health Sciences, University of Malta, Msida, Malta
e-mail: noel.abela@um.edu.mt

concluded that this was transmission of the disease from the mortuary room, as the medical students were not washing their hands when they were attending women in labour [2].

Semmelweis not only discovered the source of all evil (Fig. 11.1) but also developed a set of precautions. From mid-May 1847, large bowls of bleach stood at the entrance to the maternity clinic so that everyone who attended a birth would do so with clean hands. During the next 7 months, only 56 of 1841 women who gave birth died of maternity fever—a decrease of 3%, which was comparable to that of the midwives in the Second Department. In 1848, the figures for both departments fell to 1.2%, partly because Semmelweis demanded that the instruments used were also washed. It is still too early to discuss "disinfection" here; we have to wait over 10 years for this, until Joseph Lister developed hygienic surgery. Ignaz Semmelweis, the founding father of hygiene's motto was "Doctors, wash your hands".

Unfortunately, Semmelweis contract was not renewed. The reason for this, according to Semmelweis' own account, was that his fellow colleagues were sceptical of his results. In the end, he was marginalized and removed from his post and eventually returned to Hungary [6]. The main reason that Semmelweis failed to persuade his fellow colleagues regarding his theories was that he did not consult them with the new intervention. Today, many investigators and practitioners have learned from the error that Semmelweis made, and the "recognize-explain-act" approach is being used to improve hand hygiene compliance. Semmelweis is remembered not only as the father of hand hygiene but also as a model of epidemiologically driven strategies to prevent infection [18].

However, Semmelweis's work eventually gained recognition and has since become a cornerstone of modern healthcare practices. His advocacy for handwashing and hygiene laid the groundwork for the development of infection control guidelines and protocols that continue to save lives today. Semmelweis's legacy serves as a reminder of the importance of evidence-based medicine and the ongoing fight against infectious diseases.

He died at the age of 47 in 1865, largely unrecognized for his pioneering work in hand hygiene and infection control.

Although Semmelweis showed that hand hygiene literally saves lives, today, we are in a situation where in 2018, the ECDC published a study in which 33,000 people die every year in the European Union as a direct consequence of multidrug-resistant bacteria [3].

Fig. 11.1 Timeline of events. (Designed by the author)

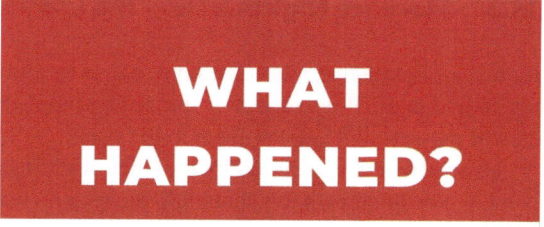

WHAT HAPPENED?

Timeline of events

Ignas Semmelweis noted that, after giving birth, mothers were dying with puerperal fever in both clinics run by Medical Students and Midwives.

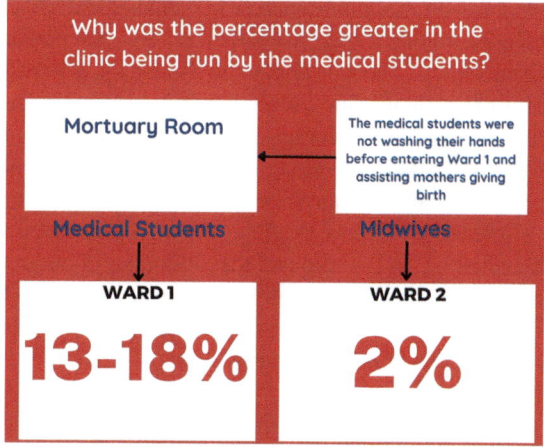

Why was the percentage greater in the clinic being run by the medical students?

Mortuary Room

The medical students were not washing their hands before entering Ward 1 and assisting mothers giving birth

Medical Students

Midwives

WARD 1

13-18%

WARD 2

2%

THE INTERVENTION

Starting today we are introducing a mandatory wash after dissections, before anyone proceeds to the maternity ward

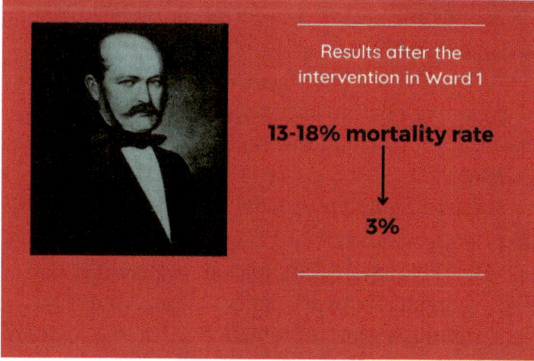

Results after the intervention in Ward 1

13-18% mortality rate

3%

11.3   Florence Nightingale—The Lady with the Lamp

Florence Nightingale, although born into a wealthy English family, she preferred not to live in an elite circle, but she decided to dedicate her life to nursing, taking care of patients and helping them to get better.

Among the famous quotes by Florence Nightingale, one finds "The first requirement in a hospital is that it should do the sick no harm."

If we look at today's situation on healthcare-associated infections, the ECDC published a press release in May 2024, where it states that each year, 4.3 million patients in hospitals within the EU/EEA are suffering from these infections [5].

Florence Nightingale published a book with the name "Notes on Nursing" 13 years after the theses of Ignas Semmelweis on hand hygiene. In these notes, she emphasized the importance of personal cleanliness. She was the pioneer and voice of nurses with respect to patient safety and prevention of infections. During the Crimean war, she was appointed to manage a British army hospital with a capacity of 4000 patients. She succeeded in improving hygiene measures, which translated into decreasing the mortality rate among the troops from 22.7% to 2.5% despite the various challenges, among them being overcrowding, outdated structure, uncaring physicians and bureaucratic inertia [4].

Although Florence Nightingale worked as a nurse during the 1860s, her recommendations on hygiene and the wellbeing of patients are still valid and are used in nursing, infection prevention and hospital epidemiology.

Nightingale's emphasis on cleanliness and hygiene laid the foundation for modern infection control practices.

11.4   Future Perspective of Hand Hygiene in Healthcare

Hand hygiene is a fundamental aspect of infection control and prevention in healthcare settings and everyday life. It involves practices that aim to reduce the transmission of harmful pathogens from one person to another, primarily through handwashing or the use of hand sanitizers.

The World Health Organization (WHO) launched the Five Moments of hand hygiene in 2009.

Although the Five Moments have been implemented worldwide and awareness of hand hygiene has increased significantly, compliance is still suboptimal across different professions and between high-income and low-income countries (64.5% vs 9.1%) [7].

The five moments of hand hygiene have been accepted by all healthcare institutions worldwide; however, in a paper titled "The Problem with 'My Five Moments for Hand Hygiene,'", Gould et al. [8] asserted that it is not always feasible to use the Five Moments for every patient all the time. The needs of patients vary greatly, and they are in a variety of situations. The Five Moments are not designed to accommodate these large variations and may even ignore obstacles that could lower hand hygiene adherence [9].

These five moments could be augmented by other actions, such as campaigns that need to be periodically refreshed, introduce non-touch technology (e.g., automatic doors), increase the frequency of environmental cleaning, especially high-touch surfaces, and rewrite hand hygiene guidelines involving both health care workers' and patients' points of view [8].

11.5 Sustaining and Improving Hand Hygiene Through Positive Deviance—Is It a Solution for Improving Hand Hygiene in Healthcare Institutions?

Healthcare-associated infections remain challenging throughout healthcare institutions, and new innovations that might increase hand hygiene compliance, which eventually results in fewer healthcare-associated infections and decreased mortality and morbidity rates, are needed.

The problem with the consistent upkeep of hand hygiene is to sustain behaviour change, as even Ignas Semmelweis wrote in his personal diary "… but to keep it up year after year, that's what I can't manage".

Positive deviance can be an alternative approach that could help improve hand hygiene compliance amongst healthcare workers and in turn result in improved patient safety.

11.5.1 Background History of Positive Deviation

Positive deviance was discovered by Jerry and Monique Sternin. In their book "The Power of Positive Deviance: How Unlikely Innovators Solve the World's Toughest Problems," they share real stories where positive deviance was implemented and translated into success stories such as childhood malnutrition, sex trafficking of girls and poor infant health [19].

Positive deviance has been used in various healthcare settings to improve hand hygiene compliance and reduce bloodstream infections in an outpatient haemodialysis unit while also reducing methicillin-resistant *Staphylococcus aureus* infections [14].

The PD approach is distinct from other popular ways to solve problems in that it imports external "best practices" but instead looks for internal answers that come from the staff within a unit. By identifying the behavioural patterns of positively deviant people in a society, the PD method creates a social network that gradually disseminates and puts these patterns into practice. This method is predicated on the idea that, despite encountering more obstacles and having access to the same resources as their peers do, there exist individuals or groups in every community whose unique behaviours and approaches allow them to develop better solutions to issues than their peers do [9].

Cohen et al. [9] presented a methodological technique in this qualitative study that can be utilized methodically at all levels, from the individual to the organization.

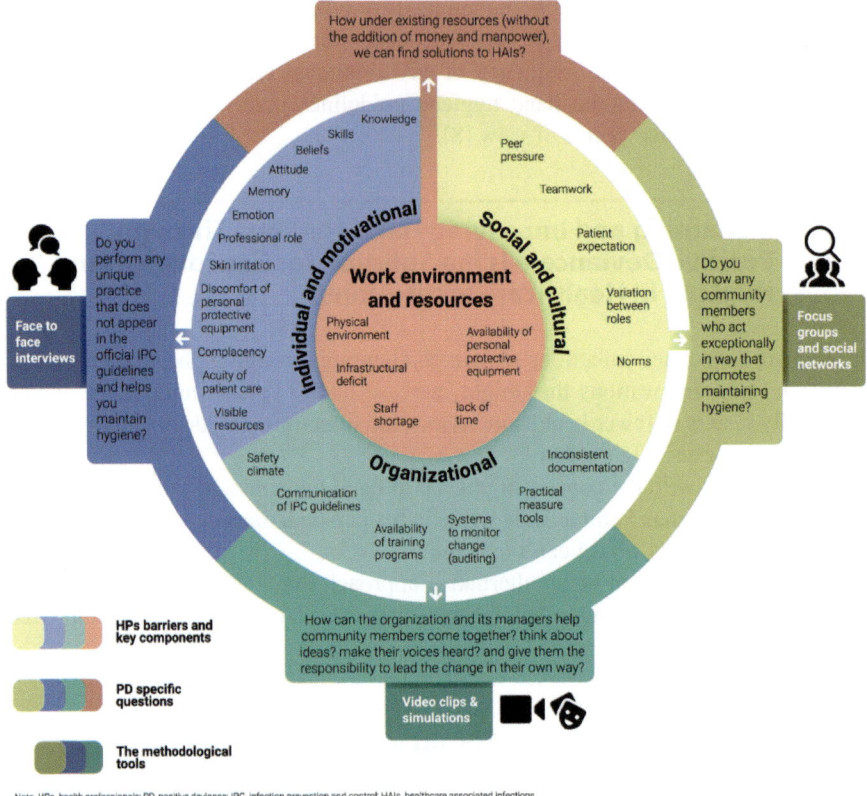

Fig. 11.2 Applied PD tool—© 2022 Cohen et al. (Published in open access article under the terms of the CC BY 4.0 License)

This illustrates how the PD approach challenges the conventional way of thinking. Instead of starting at the organizational level, it starts by looking at individual barriers before concentrating on what functions within the range of resources that are accessible. As a result, it is conducive to growth at the organizational and community levels (Fig. 11.2). By considering the obstacles identified in the literature and offering solutions, the PD approach presents a comprehensive picture of the issue and all of its nuances.

There are a number of articles about the use of positive deviance to improve hand hygiene [10–13].

When positive deviance was used as a single intervention, it improved hand hygiene compliance because PD helped create a sense of ownership among healthcare workers and highlighted that it is the most important tool for decreasing healthcare-associated infections [13]. More information on positive deviance can be found on the PDI website o (www.positivedeviance.org) [15].

Infection control personnel may strengthen their relationship with healthcare workers by identifying positive deviants involved in infection prevention and empowering their ideas to implement infection control processes. Furthermore, these ideas, which are shared by positive deviants, may be used to improve patient safety. Every day, positive deviance strives to make processes better by examining workflows, raising potential errors, and advocating for the idea that each task is both minor and crucial to the outcome. The process of learning together, assigning tasks to one another, exchanging ideas and knowledge, and evaluating each task and action continues to improve [14].

Positive deviance implementation reduces costs, which is one of the main benefits for healthcare facilities looking to increase hand hygiene compliance. Healthcare facilities have employed positive deviance to reduce MRSA infections, and the outcomes of these interventions have been excellent [16, 17].

Positive deviance is especially a possible solution to improve hand hygiene compliance in countries with low resources, as the costs of implementing it are significantly lower than those of other proposed techniques.

11.5.2 Implementing Positive Deviance in a Healthcare Facility

Positive deviance has a five-step cycle (Fig. 11.3)

1. The first step is to define the problem or opportunity, and the outcome of the intervention sought.
2. The second step is to explore the determination of unusual behaviours and practices that might help some healthcare professionals perform better than others do in their place of work.
3. The third step is creating interventions that make the new behaviours accessible to others and keeping track of the outcomes.
4. The fourth step is to design interventions so that these interventions will be accessible to others within the organization.
5. The fifth step involves monitoring the results of the intervention.

Fig. 11.3 Positive deviance cycle. (Adapted from Ref. [16])

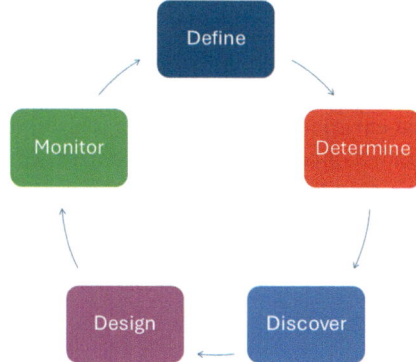

The study by Escobar et al. planned the PD intervention on these five steps, and the first step involved organizing a preliminary meeting with diverse staff members, including healthcare workers, administrative staff, community representatives and other participants. These individuals were invited to take part in this meeting on a voluntary basis to discuss and share the topics that were in review.

The topic under review was MRSA-HAI, and the group that took part in the discussion highlighted the need for improvements in existing infection prevention and control measures, e.g., hand hygiene and patient isolation.

After the preliminary meeting, a PD implementation team was set, and its target was to reduce the number of MRSA infections to zero.

The PD implementation team was trained on how to organize and manage the Discovery and Action Dialogues. The Discovery and Action Dialogues help identify and find new solutions to the problems and behaviours they are encountering by providing space to the positive deviants invited for DAD sessions to share their ideas and find better solutions than their peers do.

There are various video clips on YouTube providing examples on how to run and manage such DADs. One can watch an example of Discovery and Action Dialogues focus group at the following YouTube link https://youtu.be/zonSdYOq4pU?si=e1L iUlIsVY6Rbypp.

The main aim of the DADs sessions is to focus on the solution rather than on the problem. The PD implementation team organized 200 DAD groups and, eventually, when there was an outbreak of infections or increased healthcare care-associated infections.

After these DAD groups, the interventions chosen were as follows:

1. All patients admitted to intensive care units and those who were found to be positive were screened until they were discharged.
2. All patients in intensive care had to be washed with chlorhexidine gluconate-impregnated cloths.
3. Improvement in the oral hygiene of all patients in the intensive care unit who were intubated.

After these interventions, there was a significant decrease in the number of MRSA-HAI infections in the ICU from 1.64 to 0.62/1000 patient-days.

This study revealed that healthcare facilities that fail to reduce healthcare-associated infections with other interventions can attempt positive deviance because of its low cost and, above all, address the inclusion of all healthcare workers, create an environment for change, a transition from knowledge to sustained action, elimination of barriers to achieve adherence, and culture change.

11.6 Positive Deviance Approach—Methods Used to Implement It

While research has indicated that positive deviance can serve as a substitute strategy for enhancing hand hygiene compliance in the event that other approaches prove ineffective, positive deviance employs a bottom-up methodology that involves identifying and learning from individuals who exhibit exceptional performance on an outcome of interest. However, the methodology and procedures employed in the 37 articles that fulfilled the inclusion criteria in their systematic review were not well defined.

However, the authors noted in their assessment that the positive deviance approach still has great potential to improve the quality of healthcare, as solutions are likely to be: feasible within the current resources, staff-acceptable and sustainable [20].

In a recent article, Dhital et al. [21] applied the four steps/stages identified in the systematic review of Baxter et al. [20], which were originally adapted from Bradley et al. [22].

Framework (Steps) for the Positive Deviance Approach (Adapted from Bradley et al. [22])
1. Find "positive deviants," or organizations that regularly exhibit extraordinarily high performance in a specific field.
2. Review organizations accurately, utilizing qualitative techniques to produce theories regarding procedures that enable them to reach optimal performance.
3. Study the derived theories through more extensive, representative sampling of organizations.
4. Collaborate with important parties, such as prospective users, to spread the word about recently identified best practices.

The purpose of the study by Dhital et al. [21] was to investigate positive deviance features in front-line healthcare providers in Nepal in the early stages of the COVID-19 epidemic. This study used grounded theory methodology in its qualitative research. In-depth interviews with the 17 participants were used to gather the data; they represented various health workforce cadres and health facilities across Nepal.

The findings are structured around four major themes: challenges, finding solutions and innovations, positive lessons, and motivation. The personal challenges included fear and anxiety about the uncertainties. The professional challenges included stigma, infection control and changing work styles with the use of personal protective equipment. Despite these challenges, they managed available resources and innovated low-cost, technological and practice-based solutions. They were able to reflect upon the positive lessons learned, such as self-sustainability, teamwork, policy direction and research and self-reflection on personal growth and patient care. The intrinsic motivation included their inherent value system, and the extrinsic motivation included appreciation and acknowledgement, family and social support, psychosocial support from peers and support from higher authorities.

11.7 Conclusion

Healthcare facilities have employed various strategies to increase hand hygiene compliance, aiming to ensure that healthcare workers adhere to hygiene protocols, especially before and after patient contact. This chapter explores the historical context of hand hygiene, focusing on how Ignaz Semmelweis and Florence Nightingale succeeded in elevating hygiene standards within their respective institutions. Despite facing skepticism from their peers, their recorded data on infections clearly demonstrate that the interventions they implemented led to a significant reduction in morbidity and mortality rates. Additionally, this chapter examines the implementation of the positive deviance approach in healthcare settings to improve hand hygiene compliance. Positive deviance, which is particularly effective in low-resource settings, is a cost-efficient alternative to other interventions such as hand hygiene audits and automatic monitoring systems. Various studies from different countries have shown how the positive deviance approach has successfully enhanced hand hygiene practices and reduced hospital-acquired infections. While positive deviance shows great promise, further research is necessary, and it is hoped that future studies will continue to contribute valuable insights into improving hand hygiene compliance.

References

1. Best M, Neuhauser D. Ignaz Semmelweis and the birth of infection control. Qual Saf Health Care. 2004;13(3):233–4. https://doi.org/10.1136/qhc.13.3.233.
2. Didier P, Benedetta A. Preventing sepsis in healthcare—200 years after the birth of Ignaz Semmelweis. Euro Surveill. 2018;23(18):pii=18-00222. https://doi.org/10.2807/1560-7917. ES.2018.23.18.18-00222.
3. ECDC. 33000 people die every year due to infections with antibiotic-resistant bacteria. European Centre for Disease Prevention and Control; 2018.
4. Martischang R, Peters A, Reart AN, Pittet D. The voice of nurses in hospital epidemiology and infection control: an example from the 19th century. Int J Infect Dis. 2020;96:119–20.
5. ECDC 2024. Each year, 4.3 million patients in hospitals in the EU/EEA are affected by healthcare-associated infections [Internet]. www.ecdc.europa.eu. 2024. Available from: https://www.ecdc.europa.eu/en/news-events/each-year-43-million-patients-hospitals-eueea-are-affected-healthcare-associated
6. Jadraque PP, Carter KC. What happened at Vienna's allgemeines krankenhaus after Semmelweis's contract as assistant in the first maternity division was terminated? Epidemiol Infect. 2017;145(10):2144–51. https://doi.org/10.1017/s0950268817000875.
7. World Health Organization. Hand hygiene [Internet] wwwwhoint 2022. Available from: https://www.who.int/teams/integrated-health-services/infection-prevention-control/hand-hygiene
8. Gould D, Purssell E, Jeanes A, Drey N, Chudleigh J, McKnight J. The problem with "My five moments for hand hygiene". BMJ Qual Saf [Internet]. 2021;31(4):322–6. Available from: https://qualitysafety.bmj.com/content/early/2021/07/14/bmjqs-2020-011911

9. Cohen R, Gesser-Edelsburg A, Singhal A, Benenson S, Moses AE. Translating a theory-based positive deviance approach into an applied tool: mitigating barriers among health professionals (HPs) regarding infection prevention and control (IPC) guidelines. Thet Wai K, editor. Plos One. 2022;17(6):e0269124.

10. Marra AR, Reis Guastelli L, Pereira de Araújo CM, Saraiva dos Santos JL, Filho MAO, Silva CV, et al. Positive deviance: a program for sustained improvement in hand hygiene compliance. Am J Infect Control. 2011;39(1):1–5.

11. De Macedo R, Oliveira Jacob EM, da Silva VP, Santana EA, de Souza AF, Gonçalves P, et al. Positive deviance: using a nurse call system to evaluate hand hygiene practices. Am J Infect Control. 2012;40(10):946–50.

12. Marra AR, Noritomi DT, Westheimer Cavalcante AJ, Sampaio Camargo TZ, Bortoleto RP, Durao Junior MS, et al. A multicenter study using positive deviance for improving hand hygiene compliance. Am J Infect Control. 2013;41(11):984–8.

13. Alzunitan MA, Edmond MB, Alsuhaibani MA, Samuelson RJ, Schweizer ML, Marra AR. Positive deviance in infection prevention and control: a systematic literature review. Infect Control Hosp Epidemiol. 2020;43(3):358–65. https://doi.org/10.1017/ice.2020.1256.

14. Marra AR, Pavão dos Santos OF, Cendoroglo Neto M, Edmond MB. Positive deviance: a new tool for infection prevention and patient safety. Curr Infect Dis Rep. 2013;15(6):544–8.

15. Positive Deviance Collaborative. Positive deviance collaborative [Internet]. Positive Deviance Collaborative 2019. Available from: https://positivedeviance.org/

16. Escobar NMO, Márquez IAV, Quiroga JA, Trujillo TG, González F, Aguilar MIG, et al. Using positive deviance in the prevention and control of MRSA infections in a Colombian hospital: a time-series analysis. Epidemiol Infect. 2017;145(5):981–9.

17. AHA/Hret Guides: AHA [Internet]. [cited 2024 Oct 11]. Available from: http://www.hpoe.org/resources/case-studies/997

18. World Health Organization. Historical perspective on hand hygiene in health care [Internet]. Nih.gov. World Health Organization; 2009. Available from: https://www.ncbi.nlm.nih.gov/books/NBK144018/.

19. Sternin J. The power of positive deviance: how unlikely innovators solve the world's toughest problems. Boston: Harvard Business Press; 2010.

20. Baxter R, Taylor N, Kellar I, Lawton R. What methods are used to apply positive deviance within healthcare organisations? A systematic review. BMJ Qual Saf [Internet]. 2015;25(3):190–201. Available from: https://www.ncbi.nlm.nih.gov/pmc/articles/PMC4789698/

21. Dhital R, Subedi M, Hamal PK, Shrestha C, Bhusal S, Rimal R, et al. How positive deviants helped in fighting the early phase of COVID-19 pandemic? A qualitative study exploring the roles of frontline health workers in Nepal. Robinson J, editor. Plos Glob Public Health. 2023;3(3):e0000671.

22. Bradley EH, Curry LA, Ramanadhan S, Rowe L, Nembhard IM, Krumholz HM. Research in action: using positive deviance to improve quality of health care. Implement Sci. 2009;4(1)

Hand Hygiene: A Comprehensive Approach for Nurses

12

Camelia Bogaert

12.1 Introduction: Hand Hygiene as a Core Patient Safety Measure

Hand hygiene is globally recognized as one of the most effective measures to prevent healthcare-associated infections (HAIs). These infections exert a profound impact on patient outcomes, contributing to elevated morbidity and mortality rates, extended duration of hospitalizations, and increased financial strain on healthcare systems. According to the World Health Organization (WHO), enhancing compliance with hand hygiene protocols has the potential to reduce the incidence of HAIs by as much as 50% [1]. Such a reduction would not only mitigate the individual burden on patients but also significantly ease the operational and economic pressures faced by healthcare institutions.

From a behavioural perspective, understanding the deeper motivational drivers behind hand hygiene practices is essential for fostering sustainable compliance. Drawing on Simon Sinek's 'Golden Circle' model, which posits that effective and lasting change stems from a clear understanding of purpose—the 'why'—it becomes evident that hand hygiene must be framed not merely as a procedural task but as an ethical obligation to protect patient safety [2]. This intrinsic motivation, grounded in professional responsibility and patient advocacy, is particularly crucial in healthcare environments where patients come to heal and expect to be protected—not exposed to additional risks. Ensuring a safe, hygienic setting is not only a matter of best practice but a core expectation of professional care [9, 10]. Yet, motivation and intention alone are not enough. Sustained hand hygiene requires more than individual commitment—it depends on a supportive infrastructure. The WHO's Multimodal Hand Hygiene Improvement Strategy (MMIS) brings together essential elements

C. Bogaert (✉)
Department of Infection Prevention and Control, AZ Sint Lucas, Ghent, Belgium
e-mail: camelia.bogaertmiclaus@azstlucas.be

such as education, leadership, monitoring, and feedback into one integrated framework [4, 5].

12.2 The WHO Multimodal Improvement Strategy: A Structured Approach to Hand Hygiene

The WHO MMIS consists of five interconnected elements—system change, training and education, evaluation and feedback, reminders in the workplace, and institutional safety climate—and each element plays a vital role in embedding hand hygiene into the daily rhythm of clinical care [5].

This framework is not only comprehensive but also deeply practical, born from years of global experience and refined through frontline realities. It offers healthcare teams a dependable structure—clear, adaptable, and evidence-based—that can be relied on, even amid shifting organizational priorities [5]. As infection prevention teams often find themselves puzzling together bits and pieces from various interventions, it is worth reminding ourselves that we already have a solid framework at our disposal. Rather than reinventing strategies or navigating a fragmented landscape of disconnected initiatives, we should focus our efforts on helping all staff—particularly nurses—become well-versed in this model and embed it seamlessly into everyday practice [20, 25]. A well-understood and culturally embedded strategy not only fosters consistency but also supports organizational resilience in the face of high staff turnover. When hand hygiene expectations are clearly defined and universally practiced, it becomes easier to maintain continuity, stability, and a shared sense of purpose, even as new professionals join the team [27]. The strength of a multimodal strategy lies in the ability to bridge policy and practice, transforming best practices from abstract ideals into tangible, habitual behaviours that shape a culture of care [3]. This alignment not only enhances quality but also contributes to long-term sustainability, with evidence showing that well-integrated models can help preserve continuity and impact even during periods of staff transition or high turnover [27].

12.2.1 System Change: Build It

Laying the foundation for effective hand hygiene begins with the physical and organizational structures that support it. Ensuring that essential tools—such as alcohol-based hand rub (ABHR), soap, clean running water, and functioning sinks—are readily and reliably accessible at all points of care is a non-negotiable prerequisite for effective hand hygiene [8, 18]. These elements must not only be present but thoughtfully positioned at the point of care, embedded into the workflow in ways that promote intuitive and effortless use [15]. Evidence confirms that making ABHR dispensers more accessible in strategic, high-traffic areas leads to increased usage and better adherence [18, 23].

Yet, building a culture of compliance requires more than bricks and dispensers. The 'system' in 'System Change' must also include people—specifically, the structure of human resources that underpins infection prevention measures.

Adequate staffing is essential: when staffing levels are too low, hand hygiene opportunities are easily missed, and the ability to remain attentive to hand hygiene requirements diminishes. Dedicated infection prevention link nurses serve as integral members of the care team, acting as essential bridges between the infection prevention and control (IPC) teams and clinical services. Their role in translating strategy into action, flagging gaps, and mentoring peers is irreplaceable [19, 20].

Leadership support is another cornerstone of sustainable system change. Without visible, ongoing endorsement from management, even the best infrastructure and personnel may fall short. The commitment to provide sufficient resources and to prioritize hand hygiene at the highest levels of leadership sends a powerful signal that this is not optional—it is fundamental [20, 25].

In sum, the physical and human elements of hand hygiene infrastructure must be consistently and reliably in place across all settings and shifts. Only when these foundational conditions are met can we begin to build—and expect to sustain—a culture where hand hygiene is truly a second nature [5, 11].

12.2.2 Education and Training: Teach It

Hand hygiene education is more than a box-ticking exercise; it is an act of professional empowerment and patient advocacy. Through meaningful, evidence-based instruction guidelines, healthcare professionals gain the knowledge, confidence, and practical awareness to recognize and act according to the key hand hygiene moments. At the heart of this instruction these guidelines lies the WHO's '5 Moments for Hand Hygiene' framework [6], which provides a clear and universal structure for identifying high-risk moments of microorganisms transmission:

Before touching a patient
Before clean/aseptic procedures
After body fluid exposure risk
Before clean/aseptic procedures
After touching patient surroundings

These five moments must become second nature—not through passive learning or rote memorization, but through immersive and reflective education strategies. Simulation-based training (SBT) and role-specific e-learning modules have proven effective in anchoring these behaviours [24]. Platforms that invite multidisciplinary participation and foster dialogue across professions can also reinforce the shared accountability for infection prevention [20, 21].

Nurses, in their dual roles as learners and educators, are instrumental in bringing these strategies to life. They deliver bedsides teaching model behaviour and serve as key facilitators of hand hygiene education during onboarding, continuing education, and informal peer learning [19, 21]. Crucially, they also extend this role to patients and families—translating technical protocols into simple, empowering messages. When a patient asks, 'Did you clean your hands?' they are not undermining professional authority—they are participating in it [11, 19, 30]. This dynamic, built on mutual respect and transparency, transforms hand hygiene from a solitary act into a shared responsibility. In this way, patient partnership becomes a powerful lever for behavioural change and safety culture reinforcement [17, 20].

12.2.3 Evaluation and Feedback: Check It

Sustained behaviour change hinges on well-structured, meaningful feedback. Without timely and relevant assessment, even the most engaged healthcare professionals risk slipping into ineffective routines [4]. While traditional direct observation remains a foundational tool, it is limited by observer bias and the Hawthorne effect, where behaviour temporarily improves simply due to being watched [22].

Modern approaches enhance this foundation with electronic monitoring and real-time feedback systems that provide objective, continuous, and actionable data [8]. Digital dashboards, in particular, allow teams to visualize compliance trends and pinpoint areas for targeted improvement [7]. Wearable sensors and badge-based tracking systems can further increase visibility, offering individualized compliance insights and targeted feedback that reinforce hand hygiene habits [15, 18]. These systems, when thoughtfully implemented, support behavioural reinforcement without creating a disciplinary atmosphere. Still, the true value of these technologies lies not in the data alone, but in how that data is interpreted, communicated, and integrated into practice. Technology should not become a distant or intimidating monitor, but rather a catalyst for engagement—fuelling peer conversations, stimulating curiosity about patterns, and empowering healthcare workers to connect compliance with tangible patient safety outcomes [12].

Nurses play a pivotal role in this process. As both recipients and facilitators of feedback, they are essential to unlocking the potential of performance data. IPC link nurses, in particular, can serve as local champions who demystify dashboards, support peers in interpreting trends, and work collaboratively to identify the root causes of non-compliance. When feedback is paired with coaching and peer mentoring, it builds trust, enhances learning, and establishes a strong foundation for sustainable improvement [13].

Crucially, feedback moments must be structured and sensitively timed to ensure their maximum effectiveness [27]. Feedback should be integrated into the short- and long-term planning cycles of the IPC teams and delivered on several interconnected levels. At the individual level, it is essential during onboarding and refresher training, where new or returning staff members shape their habits and align with institutional standards. At the team level, feedback gains momentum in reflective quality huddles, regular debriefs, and peer-to-peer coaching—where open discussion and shared accountability foster group cohesion and engagement [17]. To be truly effective, feedback must be delivered when teams are psychologically ready to receive it—not during hectic clinical peaks, shift changes, or in emotionally charged situations. Misjudged timing can undermine even the most constructive message and erode trust. Choosing the right moment with emotional intelligence is as critical as the content of the feedback itself [21, 28].

Equally important are well-prepared plenary sessions, where teams present their progress, challenges, and ward-specific developed solutions to the broader hospital audience. These sessions encourage cross-learning, nurture professional pride, and strengthen team identity [20, 24]. They are most effective when attended by both clinical and managerial leadership, who by their presence signal that hand hygiene is not just a protocol, but a shared organizational priority that warrants visibility and recognition [3, 25].

12.2.4 Reminders in the Workplace: Sell It

In the dynamic and often demanding environment of clinical care, hand hygiene is a critical action that can be unintentionally overlooked. This is where strategic, well-designed reminders play a vital role. Whether presented through posters, floor decals, digital prompts, or screen savers, these visual interventions serve as gentle yet persistent nudges that keep hand hygiene top of mind in the midst of competing clinical priorities [13].

However, the effectiveness of reminders is not inherent in their presence—they must evolve to remain relevant and impactful. Static or outdated visuals risk blending into the clinical background, eventually becoming *wallpapers*—seen but no longer consciously registered [3, 12]. To preserve their communicative value, reminders must be refreshed periodically, not only in appearance but in resonance with the clinical context and routines.

While nurses offer essential insights into workflow and behavioural patterns, they cannot bear the responsibility of designing communication materials alone. This is where interprofessional collaboration is crucial. IPC teams, equipped with insights from audits, compliance observations, and ward-level feedback, should partner with institutional graphic design and communication departments. This collaboration ensures that visual materials are not only professionally crafted and targeted but also behaviourally informed and context-sensitive. Through this structured approach, reminders become more than visuals—they evolve into strategic tools for change, sustainable in both form and function [1, 9].

Each year, the 5th of May—World Hand Hygiene Day—presents a valuable opportunity to reinvigorate local engagement and strengthen institutional commitment to hand hygiene [1, 26]. However, in practice, maintaining momentum and enthusiasm for this day can prove challenging. Campaign fatigue is a well-recognized phenomenon, particularly in environments saturated with repeated messaging and stretched resources [3]. After years of repetition, the key challenge lies in ensuring hand hygiene messaging remains fresh, relevant, and emotionally resonant. Success in this space increasingly depends on creativity, inclusivity, and co-creation: leveraging storytelling, gamification, ward-based competitions, or visually compelling art installations that reflect the identity and values of each team [16]. These dynamic, participatory approaches not only refresh awareness but build deeper emotional connection and engagement with the goal of safe care [9, 25, 28]. Most importantly, they turn passive messaging into lived experience—reminders that are not just seen, but shared, discussed, and celebrated.

Authenticity and alignment with clinical realities are key. A dynamic hand hygiene culture is not built on posters alone, but on collaboration, participation, and the belief that every contribution—whether from a clinician, a cleaner, or a patient—plays a role in protecting others [24, 25].

12.2.5 Institutional Safety Climate: Live It

Embedding hand hygiene into the DNA of a healthcare organization is not merely a technical achievement—it is a cultural milestone. As the final and arguably most complex component of the WHO MMIS, this pillar emphasizes that hand hygiene must transcend protocol and become a symbol of professional integrity, mutual respect, and accountability across all levels of care [5, 28].

Living hand hygiene means more than complying with standards, it requires that strategies should be tailored. This includes adapting hand hygiene promotion to different patient populations and care contexts—accounting for cultural norms, cognitive understanding, and psychosocial factors [9, 21]. Crucially, this transformation is most successful when patients and caregivers are seen not as passive recipients but as active partners in care. Involving them in the hand hygiene dialogue—encouraging them to remind healthcare staff, modelling good hand hygiene themselves, or co-creating educational materials—deepens trust and shared responsibility [14, 30]. It repositions hand hygiene as something done with patients, not merely for them.

Yet this kind of cultural shift cannot rest on frontline action alone. Institutional leadership must visibly and authentically support the process. This includes more than policy endorsements: it requires consistent engagement with clinical teams, investment in infection prevention resources, and recognition of exemplary practices. Such leadership actions affirm that hand hygiene is a core organizational value, not a compliance checkbox [6, 20].

Finally, a mature safety climate depends on psychological safety—an atmosphere where feedback is welcomed, peer reminders are seen as support rather than judgement, and staff feel empowered to challenge norms or propose innovations. This is what allows hand hygiene to endure through periods of change or stress, and to continuously adapt as teams, technologies, and patients evolve [27, 28]. A safety climate that is lived, not merely laminated, becomes a defining feature of professional and compassionate healthcare.

12.3   The Central Role of Nurses in All Elements of the Strategy

Throughout the WHO MMIS, nurses are not peripheral participants—they are central architects of success due to their proximity to patients and insight into real-world workflows [19, 21, 27]. Across each pillar of the strategy, their contributions are both operational and transformative:

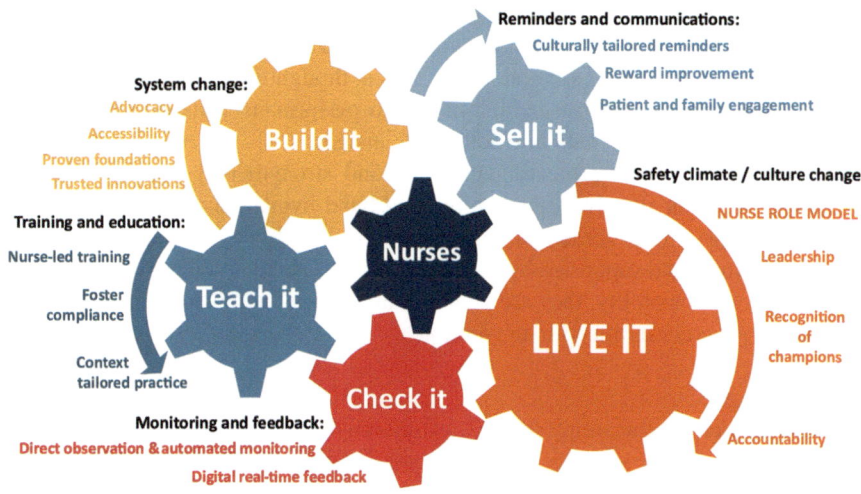

Fig. 12.1 Hand hygiene multimodal strategy. (Designed by the author adapted from WHO [5])

As system builders, they identify structural gaps and advocate for essential resources, including staffing, equipment, and workflow adaptations.

As educators, they support colleagues, mentor students, and engage patients, translating protocols into meaningful practice.

As data interpreters, they lead and learn from audits, using compliance metrics not just for reporting but as tools for collective reflection and improvement.

As communicators, they co-create and tailor workplace reminders, bridging institutional goals with clinical realities.

As culture drivers, they model safety-oriented behaviours and help embed them into the identity of the team.

Involving nurses in hand hygiene initiatives has been associated with improved compliance and a positive impact on infection rates in some studies [20, 25, 28] (Fig. 12.1).

12.4 Conclusion

Hand hygiene is not simply a task—it is a cornerstone of safe, high-quality healthcare. The WHO MMIS provides a robust, evidence-based framework to integrate hand hygiene into every layer of clinical practice. But the strategy alone is not enough. Its success depends on committed leadership, cross-disciplinary collaboration, and above all, the sustained engagement of healthcare workers at every level.

When hand hygiene becomes an integrated part of daily routines—supported by infrastructure, education, timely feedback, and visible reminders—it shifts from being an obligation to a shared professional standard. Nurses are essential to this shift: as role models, facilitators, educators, and advocates, they bring the strategy to life in real settings.

Equally vital is the role of technology. In complex and fast-paced care environments, digital dashboards, wearables, and automated systems are no longer optional enhancements—they are essential tools. When thoughtfully implemented, these technologies support staff in maintaining high performance, managing time efficiently, and transforming data into actionable insight.

Reducing infections, protecting patients, and strengthening the resilience of healthcare systems all rely in part on making hand hygiene a visible, shared, and consistently prioritized practice. Empowered healthcare teams—equipped with data-driven tools and supported by a strong culture of safety—are not only prepared to meet this responsibility; they are vital to maintaining the momentum and achieving lasting progress in infection prevention.

Key Messages

- Hand hygiene is the simplest, yet most effective tool to reduce HAIs—make it a habit.
- Be a role model—your adherence to hand hygiene encourages others to do the same.
- Ensure hand hygiene products are always within reach to boost compliance.
- Engage patients in hand hygiene—education and encouragement go a long way.
- Use technology, such as digital dashboards, to track and improve hand hygiene performance. Real-time feedback on hand hygiene compliance can lead to better infection control.
- 'Leadership is the art of mobilizing others to want to struggle for shared aspirations' [29].

References

1. World Health Organization. WHO guidelines on hand hygiene in health care: first global patient safety challenge clean care is safer care. Geneva: WHO; 2009.
2. Sinek S. Start with why: how great leaders inspire everyone to take action. Portfolio Penguin; 2011.
3. Allegranzi B, Pittet D. Role of hand hygiene in healthcare-associated infection prevention. J Hosp Infect. 2009;73(4):305–15.
4. Erasmus V, Brouwer W, van Beeck EF, Oenema A, Daha TJ, Richardus JH, et al. A qualitative exploration of reasons for poor hand hygiene among hospital workers: lack of positive role models and of convincing evidence that hand hygiene prevents cross-infection. Infect Control Hosp Epidemiol. 2009;30(5):415–9.
5. Erasmus V, Brouwer W, van Beeck EF, Oenema A, Daha TJ, Richardus JH, et al. A systematic review of studies on compliance with hand hygiene guidelines in hospital care. Infect Control Hosp Epidemiol. 2010;31(3):283–94.
6. World Health Organization. Multimodal strategies for hand hygiene improvement. Geneva: WHO; 2023. Available from: https://www.who.int/campaigns/world-hand-hygiene-day/key-resources-on-hand-hygiene

7. Sax H, Allegranzi B, Uçkay I, Larson E, Boyce J, Pittet D. 'My five moments for hand hygiene': a user-centred design approach to understand, train, monitor and report hand hygiene. J Hosp Infect. 2007;67(1):9–21.
8. Wang C, Jiang W, Yang K, Yu D, Newn J, Sarsenbayeva Z, et al. Electronic monitoring systems for hand hygiene: systematic review of technology. J Med Internet Res. 2021;23(11):e27880.
9. Arbogast JW, Moore LD, DiGiorgio M. The impact of automated hand hygiene monitoring with and without complementary improvement strategies on performance rates. Infect Control Hosp Epidemiol. 2023;44(4):638–42.
10. Pessoa-Silva CL, Hugonnet S, Pfister R, Touveneau S, Perneger TV, Pittet D. Reduction of healthcare-associated infection risk in neonates by successful hand hygiene promotion. Pediatrics. 2007;120(2):90.
11. Boyce JM, Pittet D. Guideline for hand hygiene in health-care settings: recommendations of the healthcare infection control practices advisory committee and the HICPAC/SHEA/APIC/IDSA hand hygiene task force. MMWR Recomm Rep. 2002;51(RR-16):1–45.
12. Haas JP, Larson EL. Measurement of compliance with hand hygiene. J Hosp Infect. 2007;66(1):6–14.
13. Marra AR, Guastelli LR, Araújo CM. Positive deviance: a new strategy for improving hand hygiene compliance. Infect Control Hosp Epidemiol. 2011;32(4):406–8.
14. McGuckin M, Taylor A, Martin V, Porten L, Salcido R. Evaluation of a patient education model for increasing hand hygiene compliance in an inpatient rehabilitation unit. Am J Infect Control. 2004;32(4):235–8.
15. Senges C, Herzer C, Norkus E, Krewing M, Mattner C, Rose L, et al. Workflows and locations matter—insights from electronic hand hygiene monitoring into the use of hand rub dispensers across diverse hospital wards. Infect Prev Pract. 2024;6(2):100364.
16. Apic. Two technology-based approaches that improved hand hygiene compliance are featured at infection prevention conference 2023 [Available from: https://apic.org/two-technology-based-approaches-that-improved-hand-hygiene-compliance-are-featured-at-infection-prevention-conference/.
17. Creedon SA. Healthcare workers' hand decontamination practices: compliance with recommended guidelines. J Adv Nurs. 2005;51(3):208–16.
18. Boyce JM, Laughman JA, Ader MH, Wagner PT, Parker AE, Arbogast JW. Impact of an automated hand hygiene monitoring system and additional promotional activities on hand hygiene performance rates and healthcare-associated infections. Infect Control Hosp Epidemiol. 2019;40(7):741–7.
19. Hammerschmidt J, Manser T. Nurses' knowledge, behaviour and compliance concerning hand hygiene in nursing homes: a cross-sectional mixed-methods study. BMC Health Serv Res. 2019;19(1):547.
20. Carrico RM, Garrett H, Balcom D, Glowicz JB. Infection prevention and control core practices: a roadmap for nursing practice. Nursing. 2018;48(8):28–9.
21. Monsalve MN, Pemmaraju SV, Thomas GW, Herman T, Segre AM, Polgreen PM. Do peer effects improve hand hygiene adherence among healthcare workers? Infect Control Hosp Epidemiol. 2014;35(10):1277–85.
22. Boyce JM. Hand hygiene compliance monitoring: current perspectives from the USA. J Hosp Infect. 2008;70(Suppl 1):2–7.
23. Dick A, Sterr CM, Dapper L, Nonnenmacher-Winter C, Günther F. Tailored positioning and number of hand rub dispensers: the fundamentals for optimized hand hygiene compliance. J Hosp Infect. 2023;141:71–9.
24. Meza Sierra CU, Perez Jaimes GA, Rueda Díaz LJ. Interventions to improve knowledge or compliance to hand hygiene in nursing students: a scoping review. J Infect Prev. 2023;24(1):30–44.
25. Gould DJ, Gallagher R, Allen D. Leadership and management for infection prevention and control: what do we have and what do we need? J Hosp Infect. 2016;94(2):165–8.

26. World Health Organization. Hand Hygiene Self-Assessment Framework. Geneva: WHO; 2023. Available from: https://www.who.int/teams/integrated-health-services/infection-prevention-control/hand-hygiene
27. Saito H, Okamoto K, Fankhauser C, Tartari E, Pittet D. Train-the-trainers in hand hygiene facilitate the implementation of the WHO hand hygiene multimodal improvement strategy in Japan: evidence for the role of local trainers, adaptation, and sustainability. Antimicrob Resist Infect Control. 2023;12:56.
28. Pfoh ER, Dy SM, Engineer L. The impact of hand hygiene compliance feedback on hospital-acquired infections: a systematic review. J Patient Saf. 2016;12(5):245–52.
29. Kouzes JM, Posner BZ. The leadership challenge. San Francisco: Jossey-Bass; 2003.
30. Landers T, Abusalem S, Coty MB, Bingham J. Patient-centered hand hygiene: the next step in infection prevention. Am J Infect Control. 2012 May;40(4 Suppl 1):S11–7. https://doi.org/10.1016/j.ajic.2012.02.006. PMID: 22546268.

"To Glove or Not to Glove"

13

Noel Abela

13.1 Introduction

13.1.1 Definition and Significance of Medical Gloves in Healthcare Settings

Medical gloves are single use that are used during medical interventions and examinations to prevent cross-transmission between healthcare workers, patients and the environment, especially high-touch surfaces. They serve as a critical barrier against the transmission of infectious agents and are an essential component of personal protective equipment (PPE) in healthcare settings, especially when dealing with body fluids and patients suffering from highly consequential infectious diseases.

13.1.2 Definition

Medical gloves are made from various materials, including latex, nitrile and vinyl and come in both sterile and nonsterile versions. They are designed to be worn on hands to provide a protective barrier against pathogens, chemicals and other contaminants that can be transmitted through contact.

N. Abela (✉)
Faculty of Health Sciences, University of Malta, Msida, Malta
e-mail: noel.abela@um.edu.mt

© The Author(s), under exclusive license to Springer Nature Switzerland AG 2025
B. Oomen, S. Gastaldi (eds.), *Principles of Nursing Infection Prevention Control*,
Principles of Specialty Nursing, https://doi.org/10.1007/978-3-031-84469-0_13

157

13.2   Historical Overview

13.2.1 Evolution of Medical Gloves from Ancient Times to Modern Healthcare Practices

A history of medical gloves is a fascinating journey that highlights significant advances in medical practice and infection control.

The first use of natural latex, which came from the ancient Mesoamerican Olmec culture, the oldest known major civilization in the Mexico region, occurred in 1500 BCE [1].

A detailed look at the evolution of medical gloves (Table 13.1).

13.2.2 Early History

1889: The use of medical gloves can be traced back to William Stewart Halsted, a prominent surgeon at Johns Hopkins Hospital. Halsted introduced the use of rubber gloves during surgery, not to protect the patient from infections, but primarily to protect the hands of his nurse (and later his wife) [2] Caroline Hampton, from dermatitis.

13.2.3 Development and Adoption

1890s Following Halsted's introduction, the use of rubber gloves spread slowly among surgeons. Initially, gloves were used more for the protection and comfort of healthcare workers than for infection control [2].

Early in the 1900s, the realization that gloves could also protect patients from infections began to increase traction. Surgeons such as Joseph Lister, who pioneered antiseptic surgery, recognized the benefits of gloves in reducing surgical site infections.

13.2.3.1 World Wars and Mass Production
World War I The mass production of rubber gloves began to increase, driven by the need for better protection and hygiene during surgical procedures.

World War II The demand for medical gloves has increased due to the vast number of injuries and surgeries, leading to improvements in glove manufacturing and quality control.

Table 13.1 Evolution of medical gloves—designed by author

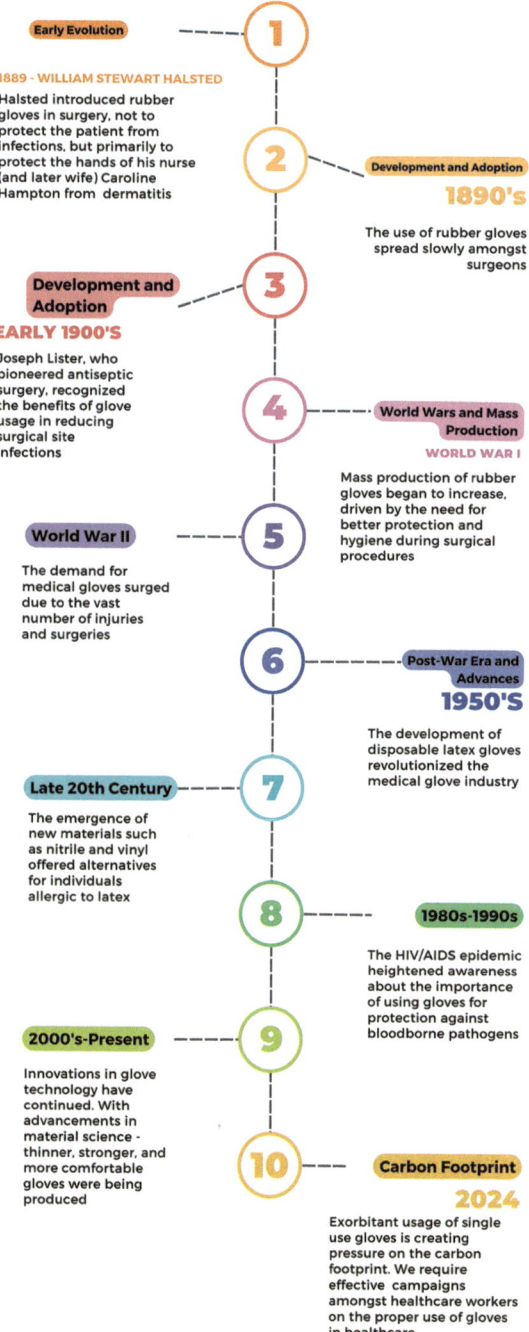

EVOLUTION OF MEDICAL GLOVES

Early Evolution — 1

1889 - WILLIAM STEWART HALSTED
Halsted introduced rubber gloves in surgery, not to protect the patient from infections, but primarily to protect the hands of his nurse (and later wife) Caroline Hampton from dermatitis

2 — **Development and Adoption**
1890's
The use of rubber gloves spread slowly amongst surgeons

Development and Adoption — 3
EARLY 1900'S
Joseph Lister, who pioneered antiseptic surgery, recognized the benefits of glove usage in reducing surgical site infections

4 — **World Wars and Mass Production**
WORLD WAR I
Mass production of rubber gloves began to increase, driven by the need for better protection and hygiene during surgical procedures

World War II — 5
The demand for medical gloves surged due to the vast number of injuries and surgeries

6 — **Post-War Era and Advances**
1950'S
The development of disposable latex gloves revolutionized the medical glove industry

Late 20th Century — 7
The emergence of new materials such as nitrile and vinyl offered alternatives for individuals allergic to latex

8 — **1980s-1990s**
The HIV/AIDS epidemic heightened awareness about the importance of using gloves for protection against bloodborne pathogens

2000's-Present — 9
Innovations in glove technology have continued. With advancements in material science - thinner, stronger, and more comfortable gloves were being produced

10 — **Carbon Footprint**
2024
Exorbitant usage of single use gloves is creating pressure on the carbon footprint. We require effective campaigns amongst healthcare workers on the proper use of gloves in healthcare

13.2.4 Postwar Era and Advances

1950s: The development of disposable latex gloves revolutionized the medical glove industry. These gloves were more hygienic and convenient than reusable rubber gloves, which require extensive cleaning and sterilization.

Late twentieth century: The emergence of new materials such as nitriles and vinyls offered alternatives for those allergic to latex. Nitrile gloves, in particular, have become popular because of their durability and resistance to punctures and chemicals.

13.2.4.1 Modern Era and Innovations

1980s–1990s: The HIV/AIDS epidemic increased awareness of the importance of using gloves for protection against bloodborne pathogens. This period saw widespread adoption of gloves across all healthcare settings, not just in surgery.

2000s–Present: Innovations in glove technology have continued, with advances in the science of clinical materials leading to thinner, stronger and more comfortable gloves. Regulatory bodies have established stringent standards for glove quality and performance.

13.2.5 Significance of Medical Gloves Today

Today, medical gloves are an essential component of personal protective equipment (PPE) in healthcare. They are used universally across a wide range of medical and nonmedical settings to prevent the transmission of infectious agents. The COVID-19 pandemic further underscored the importance of gloves in protecting healthcare workers and patients from infectious diseases.

13.2.6 Key Milestones

1889: Introduction of rubber gloves by William Stewart Halsted.

1950s: Introduction of disposable latex gloves.

Late twentieth century: Development of nitrile and vinyl gloves as alternatives to latex.

1980s–1990s: Widespread adoption due to the HIV/AIDS epidemic.

Twenty-first century: Ongoing innovations in glove materials and manufacturing processes.

The history of medical gloves reflects the continuous evolution of medical practices and the relentless pursuit of better infection control measures to ensure the safety of both healthcare professionals and patients.

13.3   Types of Medical Gloves

Latex Gloves Made from natural rubber, which offers excellent elasticity, comfort, and dexterity. However, some individuals may develop allergic reactions to latex. Today, most hospitals have switched to the use of nitrile gloves to mitigate latex allergies. However, since there are numerous items, especially single-use items, that are subsequently available, natural latex allergy remains challenging in healthcare. In some countries, gloves are produced with low allergen content or have even banned the use of powdered gloves, leading to a reduction in natural latex allergy among healthcare workers and even patients [3]. When one looks at the impact that natural latex allergies can have among nurses, it can range from 20% to 50% [3].

Nitrile Gloves Made from synthetic rubber, which resists punctures, chemicals, and pathogens and is a good alternative for those who develop latex allergies.

Vinyl Gloves Made from polyvinyl chloride (PVC), they are cost-effective and suitable for low-risk tasks but provide less elasticity and durability than latex and nitrile gloves.

13.3.1 Significance in Healthcare Settings

Protecting Healthcare Workers Gloves offer protection for healthcare workers from exposure to potentially infectious bodily fluids, harmful chemicals and other hazardous materials, reducing the risk of occupational illnesses and injuries.

Compliance with Health Standards The use of medical gloves is mandated by health regulations and guidelines, such as those from the Centers for Disease Control and Prevention (CDC) [4] and the World Health Organization (WHO) [5], to ensure safety and hygiene in medical practices.

Versatility in Medical Procedures Gloves are used in a wide range of medical settings, including surgery, dental procedures, laboratory work, and routine examinations, making them versatile PPE in healthcare settings.

13.3.1.1 Best Practices for Using Medical Gloves
Hand Hygiene Gloves should be used in conjunction with proper hand hygiene practices, including hand hygiene before and after wearing gloves.

Correct Usage Gloves should be changed between patients and different tasks to be performed with the same patient to prevent cross-contamination.

Proper Fit and Quality Ensuring that the gloves fit well and are of high quality is essential for maximum protection and comfort.

Disposal The gloves used should be disposed of according to the institution or hospital.

13.4   Raising Awareness—Glove Use Campaigns

One of the interventions that could decrease the misuse of nonsterile gloves is through awareness campaigns that need to be planned well and involve all stakeholders. Any project can take longer than anticipated, but what is important is perseverance, which is the key to success.

The aims of one of the projects [6] found in the literature were as follows:

- The staff should be encouraged to perform a risk assessment to decide whether gloves are needed for that task.
- Improving hand hygiene compliance.
- A reduction in skin allergies.
- Gloves reduce the carbon footprint of the environment.

This project was undertaken in 2016–2017 at the Great Ormond Street Hospital.

The core group consisted of infection prevention and control nurses and practice educators.

A briefing was presented, and the problems were identified. These were changes to IV drug administration and the concept of an education and awareness programme.

The following awareness programme was drafted:

- A general guideline package on when gloves should be used.
- A strategic risk assessment of when gloves should be used when preparing and administering IV medication.

The success of the programme was measured based on the following factors:

- The volume of gloves used, and the waste generated before the intervention.
- The number of staff reporting skin issues to occupational health and safety and noncompliance with hand hygiene practices were collected by performing audits in the respective wards.

The project was called "Gloves Off: Safer in our Hand". Twelve months before the launch of the project, Trust ordered 11.1 million gloves, costing £289,600. Twelve months after the project was launched, the number of glove orders decreased by 3.7 million, saving more than £90,000 to the trust.

In order for this campaign to be a success, it was important to:

- Have a clear message.
- Hold early discussions with all stakeholders.

- Align the project with what matters to staff.
- Produce graphs to demonstrate the changes.
- Refer the outcomes to staff.
- Include the communications team in dissemination.

13.4.1 Glove Use Audits

According to the literature, the use of nonsterile gloves has been associated with a decrease in hand hygiene compliance when entering a patient room or before patient contact [7, 8].

Furthermore, nonsterile gloves are used inappropriately, i.e., worn when not necessary or not changed when indicated [9–11].

The results of a study by Baloh et al. [12] that used a parallel convergent mixed method design to assess compliance rates and the gloving and HH practices of healthcare workers were similar to what has already been reported: that glove use can have an impact on hand hygiene compliance. Additionally, the healthcare workers who participated in this study said that the main reason for not performing hand hygiene before donning gloves is that they do not need to wait for their hands to dry, and they believe that it reduces skin irritation and dryness.

In our hospital, we carry out regular hand hygiene and glove use audits, observing healthcare workers with feedback on the spot.

A common practice across wards, usually observed during the period of washing patients, is going from a dirty procedure to a clean procedure while wearing the same gloves. An example of this is removing a dirty nappy and/or bedding, placing it into the appropriate bins, picking up clean bedding/nappy and returning to the patient with the same gloves. This process can continue with other elements of the washing process until the patient is ready. From speaking to staff members, the rational is "it's the same patient, so it's ok".

Double gloving for patient washing, removing one pair of gloves between the dirty and clean procedures and replacing them with a clean pair of gloves. This practice is similar to that of COVID-19 wards, which do not involve hand rubbing gloves.

Overuse/inappropriate use of gloves for cleaning practices instead of hand rubbing or washing hands.

One analysis of these observations highlights the importance of glove use awareness campaigns on the proper use of gloves among all healthcare workers.

In my experience, most of the missed hand hygiene opportunities are due to misuse of nonsterile gloves, so we need to act and try to find ways to counteract the situation that many healthcare institutions are experiencing with respect to missed opportunities for hand hygiene before patient contact.

Table 13.2 Hand hygiene compliance before and after the intervention

Contact precautions	2009 compliance (95% CI) before intervention	2012 compliance (95% CI) after intervention
Before patient contact	32.2 (24.0–40.5)	76.7 (68.9–84.5)
After patient contact	94.3 (88.0–97.9)	93.9 (89.8–98.7)
Before aseptic procedure	2.39 (14.8–32.9)	72.0 (61.6–82.4)
After body fluid exposure	56.6 (46.6–66.2)	90.9 (85.5–96.4)
After contact to patient's surroundings	No observations	90.0 (82.2–97.8)
All indications for hand hygiene	51.9 (47.1–56.6)	85.4 (82.2–88.5)

Adapted from Cusini et al. [8]

13.4.2 Glove Contamination During Use

A study by Olsen and colleagues [13] revealed that only 22% of participants recognized glove leaks after removing gloves (see Table 13.2).

The objective of this study was to test for hand contamination with gram-negative organisms and Enterococci when vinyl and latex gloves were used to perform routine procedures. Almost 64% of the gloves were found to be contaminated, and almost 25% of the leaks were identified after patient contact. The results of this study highlight the importance of performing hand hygiene after glove removal.

Alhmidi and colleagues [14] studied hand contamination after the use of gloves by applying a fluorescent solution to glove hands. Observations were made by healthcare personnel when gloves were removed using the recommended CDC technique. They also observed healthcare personnel who used the "beak" method as an alternative to the CDC recommendation. Although the CDC recommendation technique resulted in less contamination (24% vs 44%) than the nonrecommended technique did, awareness of the importance of performing hand hygiene after removing gloves among healthcare personnel is of paramount importance. An alteration of the glove removal technique can reduce contamination of the hands after removal. The suggested technique involves gripping a flap above the thumb to assist in doffing [15].

13.5 Gloves On or Off: Transmission-Based Precautions— Should We Revisit the Use of Gloves in Contact Precautions?

There is much debate regarding the use of gloves during contact precautions, which are still recommended by the WHO as part of transmission-based precautions. Recently, I was a delegate at the Infection Prevention and Control 2024 Conference in Birmingham, which was organized by Knowlex [16]. One of the speakers, Dr. Jon Otter, Director of Infection Prevention and Control, Guy's and St Thomas' NHS

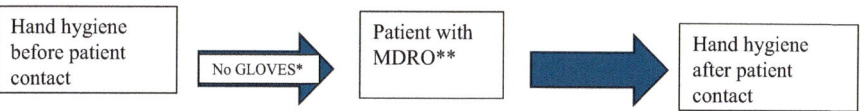

*No body fluids are present or anticipated contact with areas that are highly colonized

**Multidrug Resistant Organisms

Fig. 13.1 Use of gloves before touching a patient with MDRO. (Adapted from [16] Jon Otter presentation presented at the Infection Prevention and Control Conference held at the National Conference Centre, Birmingham 2024)

Foundation Trust, presented a presentation titled "We need to talk about gloves"; he suggested that we should revisit the use of gloves when patients are on contact precautions. He said that if a healthcare worker is dealing with a patient who is on contact precautions and has no body or anticipated contact with areas that are highly colonized, you don't need always to wear gloves provided that hand hygiene is performed after patient contact and he mentioned that we do not know the status of all our patients in the hospital who may be colonized with multidrug-resistant organisms; therefore, it makes more sense that anyone attending to patients should perform hand hygiene before and after patient contact, irrespective of their infection status by applying standard precautions. (see Fig. 13.1 designed by author).

Publications still emphasize that gloves should be used not only when dealing with body fluids but also when taking care of patients who are isolated under contact precautions [17, 18].

13.5.1 Is Hand Hygiene Sufficient to Prevent the Transmission of Infections If Gloves Are Omitted from Contact Preparations?

Jain and colleagues [19] conducted a 5-phase study on the removal of gloves in cases where there were no body fluids involved in 250 HCWs. The 5-phase study consisted of pretrial focus groups, hand microbiology, the development of a modified contact precautions poster followed by posttrial focus groups and a survey of HCWs post rollout.

During the Pretrial focus group, the central theme was "self-protection", and during the focus group, this theme was translated by the HCWs as "gloves for me—hand hygiene for the patients". The other themes were Knowledge: does not override self-protection, as they had mistrust in hand hygiene, and HCWs were task oriented, which governs their use of gloves.

In the modified contact precautions poster, they reported that gloves can be used after the risk of body fluid exposure is assessed.

In the posttrial focus groups, the central theme remained self-protection, but the theme changed from the pretrial focus groups, where the HCWs shared that "Gloves or no gloves it is hand hygiene that protects you" (see Table 13.3).

Further information that came out during the posttrial focus groups was about the revised poster.

They reported that the revised poster helped them perform a risk assessment before using the gloves, stopped their emotional response and reduced waiting time after hand rubbing.

Another theme that came out was improving patient safety, i.e., gloves are not sterile, but hand hygiene is clean and safe (see Table 13.3).

Cusini and colleagues [8] reported that after eliminating mandatory glove use, there was an increase in hand hygiene compared with that before the intervention (Fig. 13.2).

The findings of Cusini and colleagues showed that if gloves remain part of the contact precautions, compliance with hand hygiene decreases, resulting in an increase in infections among patients in hospitals. Since gloves are recommended in their institution according to standard precautions, they significantly increase hand hygiene compliance.

Table 13.3 Pretrial and posttrial themes derived from the focus groups

Pretrial focus group themes	Self-protection	Gloves for HCWs and Hand Hygiene for the patients
	Knowledge	Does not override self-protection
	Trust	They don't truly trust hand hygiene
	Task oriented	Because I am task oriented, this governs my glove use
Posttrial focus group themes	Self-protection	Gloves or no gloves, it is hand hygiene that protects you
	Visualizing	Hand microbiology results and reduction in glove waste
	Revised poster	Triggers a risk assessment for gloves, stop emotional response, and reduces waiting time after handrub
	Patient safety	Gloves are not sterile, but hand hygiene is clean and safe

Adapted from Jain et al. [18]

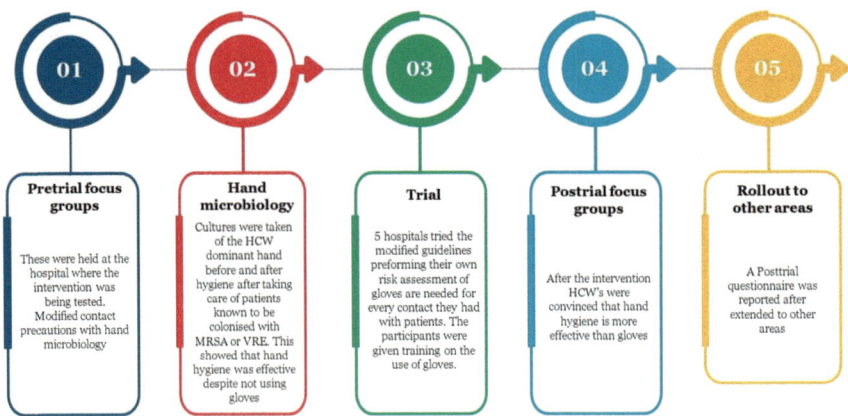

Fig. 13.2 5-phase study—modified glove use for contact precautions. (Adapted from Jain et al. [18])

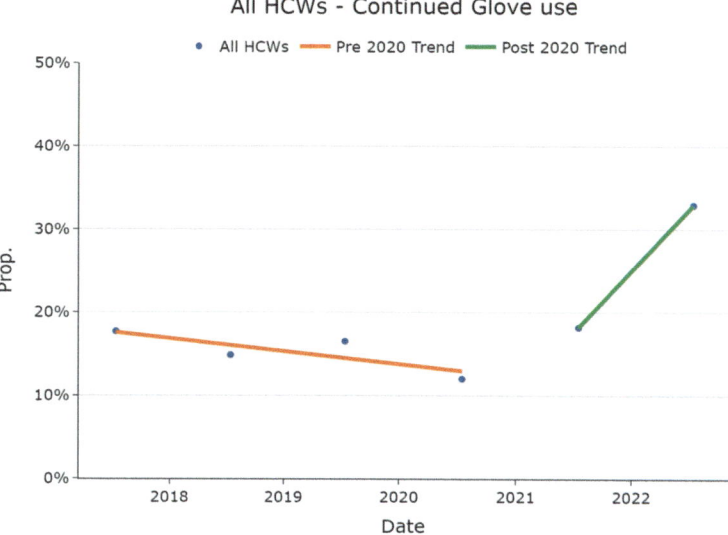

Fig. 13.3 Continuous glove use at a tertiary teaching hospital, Malta

13.6 Glove Use and the COVID-19 Pandemic

Undoubtedly, the surge in glove usage has been driven by the COVID-19 pandemic. Many infection control professionals regret that personal protective equipment (PPE) gloves are recommended for any contact with patients diagnosed with COVID-19, as this results in a decrease in hand hygiene. We know that the virus that causes COVID-19 is an enveloped virus that is fragile and can easily be killed with soap and water or alcohol hand rubs.

The hospital where I work conducts audits on glove use, and the findings of these audits indicate a considerable rise in continuous glove use both during and after the epidemic (Fig. 13.3).

In the department where I work, we have an auditor that performs audits on hand hygiene and glove use, and she has shared her personal experience with respect to glove use among HCWs, especially during the COVID-19 pandemic.

13.6.1 Healthcare Workers and Glove Use Observations by Lorraine Ellul (Hand Hygiene Auditor)

I have been observing hand hygiene and glove use for 8 years. During this time, while conducting hand hygiene audits on behalf of the infection control department, I have observed an increase in the use of gloves, particularly their incorrect use, since the COVID-19 pandemic.

I have spoken to various staff members across a range of wards to understand the reasons for wearing gloves. The feedback has varied and differs across various professions and nationalities.

Carers are the most problematic and wear gloves for all jobs because of their fear and lack of knowledge (saying "they feel safer wearing them"), and they do not understand that improper use can lead to the risk of organism transmission.

Other professionals say they wear gloves if they are uncertain about the patient's history or background and feel more secure in wearing them for any job related to the patient, protecting themselves rather than the patient or the environment.

Another reason for wearing gloves is time constraints due to staff shortages; individuals feel under pressure, leading them to cut corners and not change gloves when required to do so, which can lead to incorrect/continuous glove use.

I do highlight continued glove use issues with staff members, and the feedback is usually along the lines of "It's the same patient" after disposing of dirty linen and picking up fresh linen with the intent of making up a clean bed. Or "my gloves are clean" when staff put on gloves too soon, touching the environment before going to the patient with those same gloves. Clearly, not seeing the risk to the patient. Gloves have become a security blanket for many people, giving a false sense of security to those who choose to wear them incorrectly. I hope that with the help of future glove campaigns, we will see a positive change in the use of gloves for the safety and wellbeing of patients and the environment in which we all work.

In the literature, glove use has been associated with lower hand hygiene not only before patient contact but also when gloves are used inappropriately when patients are being cared for, such as during continuous use between patients [7–9].

13.7   The Impact of Gloves on the Carbon Footprint

The use of single gloves has increased dramatically during the COVID-19 pandemic, and this has led to an increase in CO_2 emissions, which has contributed to further pressure on climate change, where plastic has ended up in landfills that pollute the world's water systems [4].

To reduce CO_2 emissions, widespread campaigns, such as those carried out at Great Ormond Street, are needed [6].

13.7.1 Biodegradable Nitrile Gloves vs. Nitrile Gloves

Another way to decrease the CO_2 emissions produced by gloves is the production of biodegradable gloves. This approach will help to decrease the pressure on climate change. The health industry is estimated to consume 300 billion gloves annually, and it can take 100 years for a single glove to decompose [20]. In contrast, biodegradable nitrile gloves take 1–5 years to disintegrate in landfills [21].

13.8 The Future of Glove Use in the Clinical Environment

In this chapter, we have examined both the evolution of gloves in the medical field and their role in the medical field. There is already significant literature and studies, as mentioned in this chapter, that discuss the role of gloves, especially in contact precautions. We need to revisit the use of gloves in terms of infection control, costs and the impact that gloves have on the carbon footprint. Although guidelines published by the CDC and WHO still recommend the use of gloves when applying contact precautions, we need to explore whether these guidelines need to be revised, especially because robust studies have shown that omitting gloves from contact precautions does not put both the patient and healthcare workers at risk of infection [19].

References

1. Barton M. The history of surgical gloves [internet]. Past Med Hist. 2018; Available from https://www.pastmedicalhistory.co.uk/the-history-of-surgical-gloves/
2. Ellis H. The invention of rubber gloves: a true love story! | The old operating theatre [Internet]. https://oldoperatingtheatre.com/. Available from: https://oldoperatingtheatre.com/the-invention-of-rubbergloves-a-true-love-story/.
3. Bedolla-Barajas M, Machuca-Rincón ML, Morales-Romero J, Macriz-Romero N, Madrigal-Beas IM, Robles-Figueroa M, et al. Prevalencia de autorreporte de alergia al látex y factores asociados en trabajadores de la salud. Rev Alerg Mex. 2017;64(4):430–8.
4. ECDC. Use of gloves in healthcare and non healthcare settings in the context of the COVID-19 pandemic [Internet]. 2020. Available from: https://www.ecdc.europa.eu/sites/default/files/documents/Use-of-gloves-within-COVID-19.pdf.
5. World Health Organization. Glove use information leaflet Glove Use Information Leaflet [Internet]. 2009. Available from: https://cdn.who.int/media/docs/default-source/integrated-health-services-(ihs)/infection-prevention-and-control/hand-hygiene/tools/glove-use-information-leaflet.pdf?sfvrsn=13670aa_10.
6. Dunn H, Wilson N, Leonard A. A programme to cut inappropriate use of nonsterile medical gloves. Nurs Times. 2019;115(9):18–20.
7. Fuller C, Savage J, Besser S, Hayward A, Cookson B, Cooper B, et al. "The dirty hand in the latex glove": a study of hand hygiene compliance when gloves are worn. Infect Control Hosp Epidemiol. 2011;32(12):1194–9.
8. Cusini A, Nydegger D, Kaspar T, Schweiger A, Kuhn R, Marschall J. Improved hand hygiene compliance after eliminating mandatory glove use from contact precautions—is less more? Am J Infect Control. 2015;43(9):922–7.
9. Girou E, Chai SHT, Oppein F, Legrand P, Ducellier D, Cizeau F, et al. Misuse of gloves: the foundation for poor compliance with hand hygiene and potential for microbial transmission? J Hosp Infect [Internet]. 2004;57(2):162–9. Available from: https://www.sciencedirect.com/science/article/abs/pii/S0195670104001057
10. Flores A, Pevalin DJ. Healthcare workers' compliance with glove use and the effect of glove use on hand hygiene compliance. Br J Infect Control. 2006;7(6):15–9.
11. Loveday HP, Lynam S, Singleton J, Wilson J. Clinical glove use: healthcare workers' actions and perceptions. J Hosp Infect [Internet]. 2014;86(2):110–6. Available from: https://www.sciencedirect.com/science/article/abs/pii/S0195670113003812

12. Baloh J, Thom KA, Perencevich E, Rock C, Robinson G, Ward M, et al. Hand hygiene before donning nonsterile gloves: healthcare workers' beliefs and practices. Am J Infect Control. 2019;47(5):492–7.
13. Olsen RJ. Examination gloves as barriers to hand contamination in clinical practice. JAMA J Am Med Assoc. 1993;270(3):350.
14. Alhmidi H, Gonzalez-Orta M, Cadnum JL, Mana TSC, Jencson AL, Wilson BM, et al. Contamination of health care personnel during removal of contaminated gloves. Am J Infect Control. 2019;47(7):850–2.
15. UFL EHS. Glove removal technique: beak method [internet]. YouTube 2020 [cited 2024 July 19]. Available from: https://www.youtube.com/watch?v=3GvfrE4f9Ro&ab_channel=UFLEHS
16. Otter J. We need to talk about gloves [Internet]. YouTube; 2024. [cited 2024 July 19]. Available from: https://www.youtube.com/watch?v=5gWIUaiwEsQ&list=PLXw6r9VD6y_7rNLv9 rUC-TTeza4uWjUTR&index=30&ab_channel=Knowlex
17. APIC. Use personal protective equipment I infectionpreventionandyou.org [Internet]. Available from: https://infectionpreventionandyou.org/protect-your-patients/using-ppe-the-right-way/
18. Jain S, Clezy K, McLaws ML. Modified glove use for contact precautions: health care workers' perceptions and acceptance. Am J Infect Control. 2019 Mar;47(8).
19. Girou E, Chai SHT, Oppein F, Legrand P, Ducellier D, Cizeau F, et al. Misuse of gloves: the foundation for poor compliance with hand hygiene and potential for microbial transmission? J Hosp Infect [Internet]. 2004;57(2):162–9. Available from: https://www.sciencedirect.com/science/article/abs/pii/S019567010400105
20. Bruce Zou. Biodegradable Medical Gloves: The Future of Sustainable Healthcare [Internet]. www.linkedin.com. Available from: https://www.linkedin.com/pulse/biodegradable-medical-gloves-future-sustainable-healthcare-bruce-zou/
21. UC Santa Barbara. Biodegradable gloves vs. Nitrile/latex gloves: Which is better for lab sustainability? [Internet]. Ucsb.edu. [cited 2024 July 21]. Available from: https://www.sustainability.ucsb.edu/blog/just-facts-labrats/biodegradable-gloves-vs-nitrilelatex-gloves-which-better-lab-sustainability

Occupational Health and Bloodborne Pathogens

14

Tihana Gašpert

14.1 Introduction

Among health professionals, nurses frequently engage in prolonged interactions with patients while delivering care [1]. Nurses may encounter risks during interactions involving patients, one of whom is getting or transmitting an infection.

Nurses encounter the risk of harm from many sharp objects in their work environments. They typically handle injury-related items including syringe needles, lancets, surgical scalpels, cutting needles, blood collection tubes, shattered vials, razors, and scissors [2]. In healthcare environments, needle sticks and sharp injuries (NSSIs) remain prevalent; the Centers for Disease Control and Prevention (CDC) recorded over 1 million annual occurrences of NSSIs, including 8% of in-hospital injuries. Nonetheless, hardly 50% of them were documented [3]. NSSIs are characterized as any transcutaneous interaction with a sharp instrument or the penetration of a sharp object or needle that could result in exposure to blood or other bodily fluids [4].

The safety of injections is a critical concern, as injectable drugs and vaccines are frequently administered. The prevalence of needle stick and sharp object injuries among nurses worldwide varies, and although it is thought to be underreported, recent research indicates that the percentage of nurses reporting such injuries ranges from 19% to 38% [5]. Needlestick injuries (NSIs) represent the predominant occupational hazard encountered by nurses in the workplace [6]. Currently, nurses anticipate that health services will utilize over 1 million needles annually. When a nurse inadvertently punctures with a needle that has previously penetrated a patient's tissue, she is at risk of acquiring at least two possible infections [7].

T. Gašpert (✉)
University Hospital Rijeka, Rijeka, Croatia

Faculty of Health Sciences, University of Maribor, Maribor, Slovenia

© The Author(s), under exclusive license to Springer Nature Switzerland AG 2025
B. Oomen, S. Gastaldi (eds.), *Principles of Nursing Infection Prevention Control*,
Principles of Specialty Nursing, https://doi.org/10.1007/978-3-031-84469-0_14

In certain nations, the percentage of hazardous injections is 70% [8]. Engaging in dangerous injection practices, including the use of unsterilized syringes and needles, can result in a 32% transmission rate of Hepatitis B Virus (HBV), 40% for Hepatitis C Virus (HCV), and 5% for Human Immunodeficiency Virus (HIV) [8]. The World Health Organization (WHO) estimates that in 2008, unsafe injections contributed to a global burden of diseases, resulting in 340,000 Human Immunodeficiency Virus (HIV) cases, 15 million Hepatitis B Virus (HBV) infections, 1 million Hepatitis C Virus infections, 3 million bacterial infections, and 850,000 injection site infections, utilizing a probability model approach [8]. This scenario represents 14% of HIV, 25% of HBV, 8% of HCV, and 5% of bacterial illnesses globally, together with the potential to avert 28 million years of life lost to incapacity [8].

Syringe injuries are recognized as a significant source of exposure to blood-borne viruses for employees, particularly in the healthcare sector. Over 20 blood-borne viruses can be spread through infected needles or sharp objects, including Hepatitis B (HBV), Hepatitis C (HCV), and Human Immunodeficiency Virus (HIV). The probability of HIV transmission from a hollow needle injury is approximately 0.3%, whereas the risks for HCV and HBV are 3% and 30%, respectively. Globally, over 100 health workers have acquired HIV via needle injuries related to occupational hazards, along with thousands more infected with HBV or HCV. Health workers face the risk of exposure to infected blood and bodily fluids, potentially resulting in infections from HBV (Hepatitis B Virus), HCV, and HIV. Health workers and nurses frequently encounter germs that might lead to severe consequences including fatal diseases [9]. According to data from the Centers for Disease Control and Prevention (CDC), in 2002, 57 healthcare personnel were diagnosed with HIV due to exposure, including 24 nurses, while 48 officers (84.2%) were infected due to sharp items [10]. Additional research indicates that nurses experience higher infection rates due to exposure [10]. The prevalence of nurses exposed to puncture injuries from three blood-contaminated sharp items is significant. Current statistics indicate that the prevalence of needle puncture among nurses is 80.6% [10].

The standard precautions established by the CDC in 1996 are protocols designed to mitigate the risk of transmission of diseases through blood, airborne exposure, and other means inside healthcare settings. Standard care dictates that blood, bodily fluids, and secretions from patients are considered infectious materials. Standard precautions ensure adequate protection for patients and healthcare personnel in mitigating the occurrence of hospital infections [11].

A component of standard precautions is the implementation of safe injection practices [12]. Initial research conducted by investigators on various nurses suggests that their understanding of the significance of handwashing remains incomplete, and their motivation to implement safe injection practices for patients is insufficient [13]. Occurrences of work-related accidents among nurses, such as needle punctures or exposure to broken ampules, may have occurred; however, no reports have been submitted to the nursing field thus far. The nursing department head also indicated that the hospital had developed and disseminated Standard Operating Procedures (SOPs) regarding the implementation of standard precautions that nurses are required to follow [13].

Programs should prioritize the causes of NSIs. NSIs during recaps were prevalent, accounting for 16% overall [14]. Recommendations to mitigate such accidents may encompass the ban on recapping, the utilization of mechanical recapping equipment, or the implementation of a one-handed approach [14]. A recent review on the efficacy of safety-engineered injectable devices revealed moderate quality evidence indicating that these devices diminish the occurrence of needlestick injuries among healthcare professionals [15].

Adherence to standard measures, including the use of gloves and other personal protective equipment, must be reinforced through enhanced employee training. In this investigation, most healthcare workers utilized only a single pair of gloves throughout their injuries, even though donning double gloves reduces the likelihood of percutaneous exposure occurrences [16].

A Cochrane Evidence Review evaluated 34 randomized controlled trials regarding the efficacy of supplementary gloves in reducing the occurrence of percutaneous exposures among healthcare workers. Moderate quality evidence indicates that wearing double pairs of gloves reduces the chance of glove punctures and minimizes the likelihood of skin blood stains compared to wearing a single pair of gloves [14].

Prevention necessitates efficient surveillance systems. Most rely on administrative databases instead of self-reported injuries from workers, indicating poor data documentation. Nonetheless, surveillance measures are not uniformly implemented. Monitoring is essential for assessing program efficacy and for comparing alternative methodologies (e.g., discipline-specific versus generic programs). The utilization of non-disposable syringes compared to disposable and safe syringes shown a substantial decrease in preventable needlestick injuries. Furthermore, there was a notable decrease in expenses associated with the management of needlestick injuries, encompassing the psychological issues faced by workers post-injury [17].

A prevention program should be implemented in the hospital to diminish the incidence and risk of needlestick injuries among healthcare workers, as well as to mitigate the transmission of viral infections resulting from these injuries. There is a growing necessity to employ sharp devices equipped with safety engineering controls to mitigate the risk of needlestick injuries (NSIs). All healthcare workers must be taught to utilize these devices equipped with safety measures and should receive sufficient instruction on the safe handling of sharp instruments. Moreover, the recapping of needles should be prohibited, and the disposal of discarded sharp instruments must occur in designated sharps receptacles to avert damage [14].

14.2   Etiology: Causation and Implications of Disease Resulting from Needlestick Injuries

Notwithstanding the significant incidence of needle sticking in healthcare environments, most healthcare workers do not contract any infections [18]. Concerns persist over the elevated risk of disease development among healthcare workers following needlestick injuries; however, the facts do not substantiate this notion. The likelihood of a healthcare worker contracting an infection is contingent upon the type of needle, the severity of the damage, the specific organism present in the patient's blood, and the individual's vaccination history. A crucial determinant in the development of an illness is the accessibility of post-exposure prophylaxis (PEP) [18].

14.2.1 Human Immunodeficiency Virus

HIV infection is a systemic condition that predominantly undermines the immune system. Over time, nearly every organ in the body becomes implicated, resulting in a range of symptoms. The virus preferentially targets CD4 cells, resulting in a state of immunosuppression in the body. This results in the emergence of opportunistic infections, malignancies, and significant cachexia. A significant number of patients will subsequently get AIDS. Fortunately, Highly Active Antiretroviral Therapy (HAART) is now accessible, and for those who adhere to their medication regimens, mortality has become an infrequent event. Most individuals continue to lead a normal life; nonetheless, HIV remains incurable [19].

Nevertheless, the occurrence of HIV following a needlestick injury is quite rare. Only 57 of the exposed workers seroconverted to HIV. In 84% of these instances, the identified cause was a percutaneous needlestick injury. Infections acquired through exposure were 9% via the mucocutaneous route and 4% through both routes [19].

14.2.2 Viral Hepatitis

The most prevalent virus contracted from a needlestick injury is hepatitis B [19]. Approximately 30–50% of patients infected with hepatitis B may experience jaundice, fever, nausea, and nonspecific stomach discomfort. In most individuals, these symptoms will spontaneously resolve between 4 and 8 weeks. Approximately 2–5% of patients will progress to chronic hepatitis B infection. Throughout a lifetime, there exists a 15% probability that these individuals may acquire liver cancer or cirrhosis. Before the introduction of the hepatitis B vaccination, the infection rate resulting from a needlestick injury varied between 6% and 30% [19].

The management of an individual who has contracted hepatitis B due to a needlestick injury is contingent upon the recipient's vaccination status. Currently, hepatitis B virus immunoglobulin is accessible; however, its use is not advised until serological data is acquired. In unvaccinated individuals, hepatitis B immunoglobulin can avert an infection. If an individual is already infected, immunoglobulin has been demonstrated to result in a significantly milder infection. Hepatitis B immunoglobulin must be taken within 24 h post-exposure to be effective. It is utilized alongside active vaccination [19].

In unvaccinated individuals who experience a needlestick injury, the expedited hepatitis B vaccination schedule is implemented, consisting of intramuscular injections at 0, 1, and 2 months, followed by a booster at 12 months [20].

14.2.3 Hepatitis C

Healthcare practitioners are at risk of contracting hepatitis C following a needlestick injury. The precise number of healthcare professionals who have contracted hepatitis C following a needlestick injury remains indeterminate due to insufficient follow-up [19]. Epidemiological studies of healthcare workers exposed to hepatitis C by needlestick injuries indicate an infection prevalence of approximately 1.8%. Nonetheless, the current incidence of hepatitis C cases has markedly decreased. Currently, it is believed that healthcare workers who have a needlestick injury and subsequently develop hepatitis C constitute approximately 2–4% of the overall hepatitis C cases [19].

Following a needlestick injury, most individuals exhibit no signs of hepatitis C; if symptoms do manifest, they are often nonspecific and may mimic a flu-like condition [21]. In contrast to hepatitis B virus, which results in chronic infection in fewer than 6% of adults, hepatitis C leads to chronic infection in over 75% of adults. Approximately 75% of patients will develop acute liver disease, and among them, roughly 20% will progress to end-stage liver disease or cirrhosis. Approximately 1–5% of individuals will develop hepatocellular carcinoma within the following 20–30 years. Although there is no post-exposure prophylaxis for hepatitis C, certain novel pharmaceuticals have demonstrated the potential to mitigate liver damage and reduce the incidence of liver cancer [21].

14.3   Epidemiology

Notwithstanding awareness and the implementation of universal precaution protocols, needlestick injuries persist. The precise incidence of needlestick injuries remains unknown due to numerous unreported cases. Minor needlesticks are quite prevalent in the operating room. Preliminary estimates suggest that there are approximately 600,000 needlestick injuries in the US, with half remaining unreported [19]. Needlestick injuries transpire not solely in hospitals but also in various healthcare facilities, including clinics, outpatient surgery centers, day surgery units, urgent care centers, nursing homes, and cosmetic surgery clinics [19].

Needlestick injuries do not manifest with uniform frequency among all healthcare professionals. The predominant incidence of needlestick injuries is observed among nurses, surgeons, emergency medical technicians, surgical technologists, and laboratory staff. Moreover, housekeeping staff and individuals responsible for cleaning sharp containers are at significant risk for needlestick accidents [15].

14.4   Influence of Safety Devices on Needlestick Injuries

Special safety-engineered devices (SEDs) have been extensively promoted to mitigate the occurrence of needlestick injuries. Contrary to the anticipated reduction in needle sticks with increased utilization of SEDs, research indicates that the frequency of needle sticks may have risen. A 2018 study conducted in the Netherlands reported a needle stick rate of 1.9 per 100 healthcare workers before the adoption of SEDs. Following the introduction of SED, the frequency of needlestick injuries rose to 2.2 per 100 healthcare professionals. The predominant factors identified for needle sticking in the study were challenges in utilizing the safety device and ongoing inappropriate disposal of needles [22].

14.5   Improving Healthcare Team Performance

Although the majority of needlestick injuries do not result in infection transmission, there are instances where a severe, persistent infection such as HIV or hepatitis C may occur. Healthcare professionals bear the responsibility for preventing needlestick injuries first. Experts assert that no singular safety policy is universally effective; therefore, it is vital to implement a comprehensive policy that acknowledges the conduct of healthcare personnel, institutional regulations, and the safe use of sharps and other instruments. An essential component of any preventive program is minimizing needle usage wherever feasible and employing alternative solutions when accessible. Hospital personnel may also participate in ongoing education and training regarding the latest technology employed in dialysis and blood extraction. A monitoring program is crucial as it can mitigate potential risk factors associated with needlestick injuries, hence ensuring the system's efficacy. Currently, most hospitals possess an infectious disease committee of a nurse, pharmacist, laboratory technologist, physician, and risk management professional, which formulates and implements safety regulations. Nevertheless, due to the nurse's role, they are ideally situated to guarantee compliance with safety regulations. The sole method to mitigate needlestick injuries is via vigilance, strict enforcement of regulations, and conducting random audits of healthcare personnel [19].

14.6 Mitigation of Needle-Stick Injuries and Other Blood Exposures by a Hierarchy of Controls

Methods employed to mitigate occupational hazards have conventionally been addressed in terms of hierarchy arranged in order of precedence. The following list ranks injuries and other blood exposures from the most to least effective [23]:

- Elimination of hazard—The total eradication of a hazard from the workplace is the most efficient method for danger control; this strategy should be employed whenever feasible.
  - eliminating sharps and needles when feasible (e.g. by replacing needles with jet injectors) and syringes, or employing needleless intravenous systems;
  - eliminating any superfluous injections;
  - removing superfluous sharp instruments, such as towel clips.
- Engineering controls—These are implemented to isolate or eliminate a hazard from the workplace.
  - containers for the disposal of sharps;
  - if feasible, employ (sharp protection devices for all procedures involving needles that retract, sheathe, or dull shortly following usage).
- Administrative controls—These are regulations, such as Standard Operating Procedures (SOPs), designed to mitigate exposure to the peril.
- The distribution of resources indicating a dedication to the safety of healthcare personnel.
- A committee for the prevention of needlestick injuries.
- An exposure control plan.
  - elimination of all hazardous devices;
  - regular training on the utilization of safe devices.
- Work practice controls—These are measures designed to modify worker behavior to mitigate risks.
- No recapping of needles.
  - positioning sharps containers at eye level and within arm's reach;
  - sealing and disposing of sharps containers when they are three-quarters full;
  - implementing protocols for the secure management and disposal of sharp instruments prior to commencement.
- A protocol.
- Occupational hazards and management of bloodborne infections.
- Personal protection equipment.

14.7 Conclusion

Despite significant progress in the creation of safer needles and sheathing devices, these instruments are not infallible and are effective only in environments that are consistently supervised. Research indicates that the regular implementation of these needleless systems significantly reduces needlestick injuries. Currently, healthcare facilities bear the responsibility of educating and training their personnel on the safe utilization of sharps and needles. Employees must understand the ramifications of needlestick injuries and the measures that can be implemented to prevent them. Currently, most hospitals have implemented policies and practices to avert needlestick injuries by promoting the following measures:

- Develop an occupational health and safety program that primarily assesses and identifies high-risk procedures and suggests appropriate safety measures.
- Implement safe needle utilization protocols and employ needleless devices whenever feasible.
- Determine the origin of any injuries sustained and the potential preventive measures that could have been implemented.
- Reduce the utilization of needles whenever feasible.
- Promote the utilization of needles equipped with safety mechanisms.
- Modifies any hazardous work practices on the floor and in the operating room.
- Educates healthcare personnel on needlestick injuries, their prevention, and the latest management protocols.
- Fosters a safety culture devoid of retribution.
- Promote the reporting of hazardous practices without the apprehension of reevaluation.
- Performs random audits to verify adherence to hospital policies and procedures.
- Evaluate results periodically.

References

1. Scott A. Patient safety, satisfaction, and quality of hospital care: cross sectional surveys of nurses and patients in 12 countries in Europe and the United States. Br Med J (BMJ). 2012;2012(344).
2. Fadil RA, Abdelmutalab NA, Abdelhafeez SA, Mazi W, Algamdi S, Shelwy MM, et al. Pattern and risk factors of sharp object injuries among health care workers in two tertiary hospitals, Al Taif-Kingdom of Saudi Arabia 2016–2018. Saudi J Biol Sci. 2021;28(11):6582–5.
3. Musa S, Peek-Asa C, Young T, Jovanovic N. Needle stick injuries, sharp injuries and other occupational exposures to blood and body fluids among health care workers in a general hospital in Sarajevo, Bosnia and Herzegovina. Int J Occup Saf Health. 2014;4(1):31.
4. Ahmed SF, Shakor JK, Hamedon TR, Jalal DMF, Qadir DO. Prevalence of needle stick and sharp injuries among surgical specialist hospital-cardiac center in Erbil City: a cross-sectional study. Tabari Biomed Stud Res J. 2020.
5. Adefolalu A. Needle stick injuries and health workers: a preventable menace. Ann Med Health Sci Res. 2014;4(Suppl 2):S159.
6. Mahajan P, Shinde S, Pandey N, Sharma Y, Kousal V, Bavoria S. Needle stick injuries as an occupational hazard: awareness, perception and practices amongst nurses in a premier tertiary care hospital of northern India. Eur J Mol. Clin Med. 2022;9(03).
7. Mohamud RYH, Mohamed NA, Doğan A, Hilowle FM, Isse SA, Hassan MY, et al. Needlestick and sharps injuries among healthcare workers at a Tertiary Care Hospital: a retrospective single-center study. Risk management and healthcare. Policy. 2023:2281–9.

8. Gyawali S, Rathore DS, Kc B, Shankar PR. Study of status of safe injection practice and knowledge regarding injection safety among primary health care workers in Baglung district, western Nepal. BMC Int Health Hum Rights. 2013;13:1–7.
9. Efstathiou G, Papastavrou E, Raftopoulos V, Merkouris A. Factors influencing nurses' compliance with standard precautions in order to avoid occupational exposure to microorganisms: a focus group study. BMC Nurs. 2011;10:1–12.
10. Luo Y, He G-P, Zhou J-W, Luo Y. Factors impacting compliance with standard precautions in nursing, China. Int J Infect Dis. 2010;14(12):e1106–e14.
11. Haile TG, Engeda EH, Abdo AA. Compliance with standard precautions and associated factors among healthcare workers in Gondar University comprehensive specialized hospital, Northwest Ethiopia. J Environ Public Health. 2017;2017(1):2050635.
12. Van Tuong P, Phuong TTM, Anh BTM, Nguyen THT. Assessment of injection safety in Ha Dong General Hospital, Hanoi, in 2012. F1000Research. 2017;6.
13. Kusnan A, Binekada IMC, Susanty S, Hajri WS, Afrini IM, Syam Y. Safe injection practices and the incident of needle stick injuries (NSIs). Enferm Clin. 2020;30:73–6.
14. Alfulayw KH, Al-Otaibi ST, Alqahtani HA. Factors associated with needlestick injuries among healthcare workers: implications for prevention. BMC Health Serv Res. 2021;21:1–8.
15. Lavoie MC, Verbeek JH, Pahwa M. Devices for preventing percutaneous exposure injuries caused by needles in healthcare personnel. Cochrane Database Syst Rev. 2014;3.
16. Mischke C, Verbeek JH, Saarto A, Lavoie MC, Pahwa M, Ijaz S. Gloves, extra gloves or special types of gloves for preventing percutaneous exposure injuries in healthcare personnel. Cochrane Database Syst Rev. 2014;3.
17. Sabermoghaddam M, Sarbaz M, Lashkardoost H, Kaviani A, Eslami S, Rezazadeh J. Incidence of occupational exposure to blood and body fluids and measures taken by health care workers before and after exposure in regional hospitals of a developing country: a multicenter study. Am J Infect Control. 2015;43(10):1137–8.
18. Dulon M, Wendeler D, Nienhaus A. Seroconversion after needlestick injuries–analyses of statutory accident insurance claims in Germany. GMS Hyg Infect Control. 2018:13.
19. King KC, Strony R. Needlestick. Treasure Island: StatPearls Publishing; 2018.
20. Triassi M, Pennino F. Infectious risk for healthcare workers: evaluation and prevention. Ann Ig. 2018;30(4):48–51.
21. Demsiss W, Seid A, Fiseha T. Hepatitis B and C: Seroprevalence, knowledge, practice and associated factors among medicine and health science students in Northeast Ethiopia. PLoS One. 2018;13(5):e0196539.
22. Schuurmans J, Lutgens S, Groen L, Schneeberger P. Do safety engineered devices reduce needlestick injuries? J Hosp Infect. 2018;100(1):99–104.
23. World Health Organization. Prevention of hospital-acquired infections: a practical guide. World Health Organization; 2002.

Outbreak Management and Surveillance

15

David Valente Peres and Isabel Neves

15.1 Definitions

Outbreaks are adverse events that can happen in a variety of settings. When it occurs in a healthcare setting, it is the responsibility of the Infection Control Professional (ICP) to help identify, investigate the source of that outbreak, reduce its effects and prevent its recurrence. But what is an outbreak? To be able to answer this question it is important to review some epidemiological concepts first.

According to Table 15.1, an outbreak falls in the epidemic category but is more restricted in terms of time and geographical area. According to Last [2] an outbreak is "a small, localized cluster of cases of a condition, usually an infectious disease. The word is sometimes a euphemism used to downplay the seriousness of an epidemic" [2]. By cluster it is meant "an aggregation of cases grouped in place and time that are suspected to be greater than the number expected, even though the expected number may not be known" [3].

So, we can infer that an outbreak can be described as a group of cases that are linked by both time and place. These are usually suspected to come from a common source of infection. They can be:

D. V. Peres (✉)
Infection and Antimicrobial Resistance Control Department, Matosinhos Local Health Unit, Matosinhos, Portugal

Portuguese National Infection Control Association (ANCI), Lisboa, Portugal

I. Neves
Infection and Antimicrobial Resistance Control Department, Matosinhos Local Health Unit, Matosinhos, Portugal

Portuguese National Infection Control Association (ANCI), Lisboa, Portugal

Infectious Diseases Department, Matosinhos Local Health Unit, Matosinhos, Portugal

Table 15.1 Levels of disease occurrence

Sporadic	A sporadic disease occurs infrequently and irregularly amongst a population.
Endemic	Endemic is defined as "the constant presence and/or usual prevalence of a disease or infectious agent in a population within a geographic area"
Epidemic	Epidemic is defined as an increase, which is often sudden, in the number of cases of a disease above what is normally expected in that population in that area. An epidemic is typically more prolonged and widespread than an outbreak.
Pandemic	Pandemic is defined as a global epidemic that spreads in several countries or continents, usually affecting a large number of people.

Adapted from WHO—Outbreak investigations in health facilities [online course] World Health Organization, 2022

- a greater than expected incidence of infection (when compared to the usual background rate of the facility or ward);
- a single case of a rare or epidemic disease;
- a suspected, or actual, event that involves microbiological contamination of food or water (e.g., sink drains, water reservoirs) [1].

The ICP should be aware and confirm if it is really an outbreak. In fact, "pseudo-outbreaks" can occur as consequence of changes in health care practices, new epidemiological case definitions or changes in laboratory procedures or techniques.

Regardless of the source, an outbreak must be investigated, since history taught us the potential devastation of these events, which can originate an epidemic or even a pandemic. In fact, diseases such as cholera, influenza, malaria, smallpox and the plague are described as causes of epidemics and pandemics that killed millions of people and affected the lives of many others [4]. More recently, the SARS-CoV-2 infection (that originated the COVID-19 pandemic) and the Monkey pox infection are other examples [5, 6].

15.2   Competences of the ICP in Outbreak Management

In healthcare environment, infectious diseases can spread quickly among staff and patients who are more susceptible to infections, as result of their illness or treatment. Despite high standards of infection control practice, there is always the possibility of outbreak occurrence [7].

During an outbreak, an ICP can face many challenges such as lack of coordination with other teams; insufficient human resources; poor information in patient records; staff resistance to recognizing incorrect practices or to implement control measures, as well as the pressure of time. To manage these challenges, the ICP should have certain competences that can help to investigate and control the outbreak.

In 2013 the *European Center for Disease Control and Prevention* (ECDC) described, as one of the domains in the competences of ICP, "identifying, investigating and managing outbreaks", specifying the following competences:

- Identify clusters of healthcare-associated infections (HAI) through contacts with clinical units and laboratories or through alerts or systematic analysis of microbiological laboratory testing;
- Manage an outbreak of infections at healthcare organization or community level;
- Carry out descriptive and analytic investigations of the outbreak;
- Select appropriate methods of molecular typing and interpret microbiological results in close collaboration with clinical/reference microbiology laboratories;
- Formulate and implement a suitable strategy for identifying and communicating (internally and externally) with concerned actors, including those in primary, acute and long-term care;
- Interpret findings and report them to relevant people by using appropriate means and seek the relevant internal and external personnel advice;
- Use lessons learned from outbreak investigations to inform quality improvement measures [8].

More recently, in 2020, the *World Health Organization* (WHO) published its version of ICP Core competences, where, in the area "Infection prevention and control in clinical practice", there is the domain "Health care-associated outbreak prevention and management" in which the competence summary refers to "prevent, detect, manage and control health care-associated outbreaks" and "conduct or support infection prevention and control training activities and develop and/or use effective communications during outbreaks in health care facilities". To fulfil this competence, "knowledge" and "ability" items are described, subdivided in "Policy and Guidance"; "Leadership and implementation"; "Education and training"; "Communications and advocacy" and "Monitoring" [9].

Using its competences in this area, the ICP must establish the objectives when facing an outbreak, namely:

- Stop the outbreak as quickly as possible to protect patients (ensure rapid response and implement control measures that will stop the transmission);
- Maintain the public's confidence (recognizing that patient and staff safety is the primary focus and considering its impact in patient care and public perception);
- Recognize new risks associated with healthcare delivery;
- Prevent future outbreaks (identifying systemic problems and mitigating gaps in infection control) [10].

15.3 Outbreak Investigation Steps

An outbreak investigation involves many steps but not all steps may be performed in every outbreak, their order may vary, and multiple steps may be performed simultaneously. Although not specific of the healthcare setting, these steps, described in Table 15.2, are a useful guide in conducting an outbreak investigation [11].

Table 15.2 Steps in outbreak investigation

Outbreak investigation: characterization and investigation steps
1. Verify the diagnosis
2. Confirm existence of outbreak
3. Assemble outbreak management team and implement immediate control measures
4. Develop a case definition
5. Identify and search for cases
6. Perform descriptive epidemiology
7. Develop and evaluate hypotheses
8. Consider environmental assessment
9. Perform infection control assessment and implement control measures
10. Maintain surveillance and communicate findings

Adapted from WHO (2022) and King et al. (2019)

15.3.1 Verify the Diagnoses

Identification, as accurately as possible, the specific nature of the disease (by ensuring that the diagnosis is correct) is an important basic step. To do so, confirmatory laboratory tests (if available) or combinations of symptoms (subjective complaints), signs (objective physical findings) and other findings should be reviewed. This should be made to confirm the problem that was reported, to rule out misdiagnosis or potential laboratory errors and overcome the possibility of being a pseudo-outbreak [12].

Diagnoses can be confirmed by implementing the following activities:

- Interview the cases;
- Clinical examination of cases, when possible;
- Medical records review;
- Confirm the laboratory results.

15.3.2 Confirm Existence of Outbreak

As important as to verify the diagnosis, the confirmation of the presence of an outbreak is crucial, before committing program resources to a full-scale investigation. This can be difficult since there are several factors that can be confounding, namely:

- Some cases may be unrelated to the outbreak;
- Increased or changed local reporting procedures or changes in case definition;
- Increased awareness in certain agents or illnesses;
- Improvements or other changes in diagnostic procedures;
- Just a single case may be treated as a potential outbreak for response purposes if the pathogen or situation is unusual or is a sentinel event [10].

To confirm the existence of an outbreak, the number of cases during the suspected period should be compared with the number of cases that would be expected during a non-outbreak timeframe. This can be done through comparing time frames just before the suspected period (or the corresponding period from the previous year, particularly if the adverse event has a seasonal periodicity) and calculation of rates (if possible) between timeframes [12].

15.3.3 Assemble Outbreak Management Team and Implement Immediate Control Measures

Upon confirmation of an outbreak, a team should be assembled to coordinate and implement the activities of the investigation. This team should include members of the infection control team (doctor and nurse), infection control link professionals, clinical director (or his/her representative), head of the affected unit(s), chief nursing officer (or his/her representative), communication / public relations representative, microbiologist and hospital epidemiologist.

This team should be responsible for the following activities:

- Follow and actively seek new cases;
- Identify exposed patients;
- Plan and implement infection control strategies;
- Determine the outbreak etiology (if possible);
- Introduce practice improvements to prevent future outbreaks;
- Manage communication strategies [1].

Concomitantly, with the information available, it is important to put in place immediate infection control measures. Table 15.3 describes possible actions in this field.

15.3.4 Develop a Case Definition

According to WHO [1] "a case definition is a standard set of criteria established in order to determine whether an individual should be classified as having the condition of interest (…) and is initially designed to be more sensitive than specific". This means it is intended to ensure that no cases are missed, avoiding false positives (cases not correctly identified as part of the outbreak) and finding all cases that belong to the outbreak. A case definition should be dynamic, that is, it should be refined as new information is obtained, starting out as broad and then narrower, as the investigation goes on.

A good case definition should include:

- WHO: Person or affected population, e.g., age, sex, race, occupation.
- WHERE: Place, e.g., geographic location or facility.

Table 15.3 Possible immediate interventions for outbreak management

Immediate control measures for outbreak management	
Type of transmission suspected	Suggested action
Cross-transmission (transmission between persons)	Transmission-based precautions according to the infectious agent(s). Create isolation cohorts of patients. Set health professionals cohort to care of these patients.
Hand transmission	Reinforcement of good practices in handwashing and nonsterile glove use.
Airborne infections	Triage, detection and patient isolation with recommended ventilation type.
Agent present in water, waterborne agent	Assessment of water system, liquid products or medication. Use of disposable devices where reusable equipment is suspected.
Foodborne agent	Reinforcement of good practices in food handling. Elimination of the suspected food.
Environmental reservoirs	Review and enhancement of cleaning and disinfection processes. Interruption of suspected mode of delivery from environment to patient.
Colonized or infected healthcare personnel	Review of facility policies, work restrictions, duty exclusions, treatment, in collaboration in Occupational Health Unit.

Adapted from Christensen et al. (2019)

- WHEN: Time, e.g., the time period associated with illness onset.
- WHAT: Combination of simple and objective clinical features (e.g., sudden onset of fever and cough) <u>AND</u> the presence of specific laboratory findings (if applicable).
- DEGREE OF CERTAINTY: Suspect, probable or confirmed [1].

> Example of a Case Definition: A resident of, or visitor to, Rapid City, South Dakota, who was diagnosed by a physician, either clinically or radiographically, with community-acquired pneumonia with symptom onset after May 1, 2022, and who had laboratory confirmation of Legionnaires' disease by culture of *Legionella*, by urinary antigen test for *Legionella pneumophila* serogroup 1 (Lp1), by a fourfold or greater rise in serum antibody titer to Lp1, or detection of specific *Legionella* antigen by direct fluorescent antibody staining [14].

Criteria should be defined to differentiate the degrees of certainty, which can be divided as:

- Suspect (Possible): usually has fewer of the typical clinical features or weaker epidemiologic links to confirmed cases;
- Probable: usually has typical clinical features and an epidemiologic link to confirmed cases but lacks laboratory confirmation;
- Confirmed: usually must have laboratory verification [10].

15.3.5 Identify and Search for Cases

Once the case definition has been developed, search for new cases should be conducted. Identification of cases is important for several reasons: it helps investigators to confirm the presence of an outbreak, formulate hypotheses for its cause, support efforts to identify and evaluate potential risk factors and plan the resources necessary to manage the situation.

The approach to finding cases can be adjusted over time, from broad in the beginning to, in a later stage, more specific (just like in the case definition). It can be made retrospectively or prospectively. The following sources are available for retrospectively case finding:

- Laboratory records;
- Infection control surveillance records;
- Other records, for example from occupational health, pharmacy, radiology, admission/discharge or logs specific to the infection type (e.g., operating room logs to identify surgical site infections).
- Public health surveillance data (e.g., reportable condition and public health reports)
- Staff interviews [10].

On the other hand, *prospective* case identification can be done through:

- A call for cases, that is, ask health professionals, other facilities or public health agencies to recall or be alert (can be both retrospective or prospective);
- Notification of healthcare professionals to raise awareness, ensure appropriate testing, and report suspect cases to the outbreak management team;
- Notification of laboratory staff to ensure appropriate testing, report suspect cases and ensure storage of clinical specimens to ensure further testing can be performed;
- Active surveillance testing of patients at risk who may be colonized or infected with specific pathogens (e.g., rectal swab cultures to screen for carbapenemase-producing *Enterobacterales*) to identify additional cases [10].

The ICP should be aware that potentially exposed individuals may include healthcare professionals, visitors or even community residents. Healthcare professionals testing should only be done when consistent with the epidemiologic scenario and part of a plan developed together with Occupational Health to manage the positive results. This plan should include duty or work restrictions; possible decolonization or other specific control strategies to undertake for staff who test positive and possible vaccination or treatment prophylaxis (if applicable) for exposed negative ones [15].

15.3.6 Perform Descriptive Epidemiology

Descriptive epidemiology is a process that can identify patterns among cases and in populations by person, time and place. Through systematic review of the collected data, it can be possible to construct line lists or spot maps, draw epidemic curves and compare groups of individuals.

15.3.6.1 Line Lists

Information about all cases should be collected and put in a form of a list to help identify common traits and exposures. This document can be important to pinpoint the source of the outbreak and devise effective control measures [16].

Information typically included in a line list is:

- Personal identifiers: name initials, number of medical record, bed location;
- Demographic data: age, sex;
- Clinical information: at a minimum, information required to confirm that patients meet the case definition;
- Risk factors: know contacts with other cases and/ or environmental exposures, travel history;
- Laboratory results;
- Treatment received and outcome.

In Table 15.4 it can be seen an example of a line-list of KPC-producing *Klebsiella pneumoniae* outbreak at a Portuguese university hospital.

15.3.6.2 Epidemic Curve

An epidemic curve is a graph (histogram) in which the cases of disease that occurred during the outbreak are plotted according to time of the cases detection. This curve is constructed to study the epidemic pattern of the disease and helps to determine whether the source of infection is common and continuing, identify the probable time of exposure of the cases to the source of infection and probable incubation period [18].

The epidemic curve can allow an estimate of the incubation time, which can help in the identification of the microorganism. The time from the presumed exposure to the peak of the epidemic curve is the hypothesized median incubation time. The shape of the curve can, also, as shown in Fig. 15.1, give an indication of the mode of transmission and whether the infection control measures are being effective [19].

- When the number of cases rises abruptly and falls again in a log linear fashion, we are in the presence of a *point source* (the population at risk was exposed at one time).
- On the other hand, a *continuous common source* occurs where there is continued exposure of individuals and the shape of the curve rises suddenly but do not disappear because more individuals continue to be exposed to the source.

Table 15.4 Line-list of KPC-producing *Klebsiella pneumoniae* outbreak at a Portuguese university hospital

Ref.	Sex, age (y)	Diagnosis	Ward	Number of risk factors	LOS to KPC (d)	Total LOS (d)	Type of sample	PFGE clone	Infection/ colonization	Immediate outcome
1	M, 84	Bone fractures (multiple myeloma)	Orthopedics	3	31	33	Sputum	001	Infection	Died
2	M, 52	Brain tumor	Neurosurgery	5	4	43	Urine	001	Colonization	Other hospital
3	F, 84	Congestive heart failure decompensation	Medicine	7	5	24	Urine	001	Colonization	Died
4	M, 81	Aspiration pneumonia	Orthopedics/ medicine	11	0	7	Sputum	001	Colonization	LTCF
5	F, 81	Renal decompensation	Medicine	5	4	5	Urine	001	Colonization	Home
6[a]	M, 74	Peripheral arterial disease	Vascular surgery	4	97	138	Rectal swab/CVC	001	Infection	Died
7	M, 55	Peripheral arterial disease	Vascular surgery	0	26	52	Rectal swab	No info[b]	Colonization	Home
8	M, 69	Peripheral arterial disease	Vascular surgery	1	19	44	Rectal swab	No info[b]	Colonization	LTCF
9	M, 80	Peripheral arterial disease-infected toes	Vascular surgery	3	52	79	Rectal swab/ Wound	001	Infection	Home
10	M, 84	Prosthesis infection	Vascular surgery	4	12	14	Rectal swab/ Wound	001	Colonization	Home

Reproduced from Ref. [17]

ASC active surveillance culture (rectal swab), *CVC* central venous catheter, *F* female, *KPC-Kp* KPC-producing *Klebsiella pneumoniae*, *LOS* length of stay, *LTCF* long-term care facility, *M* male, *PFGE* pulsed field gel electrophoresis

[a]Index case

[b]Impossibility to send these samples to molecular analysis because of logistic reasons

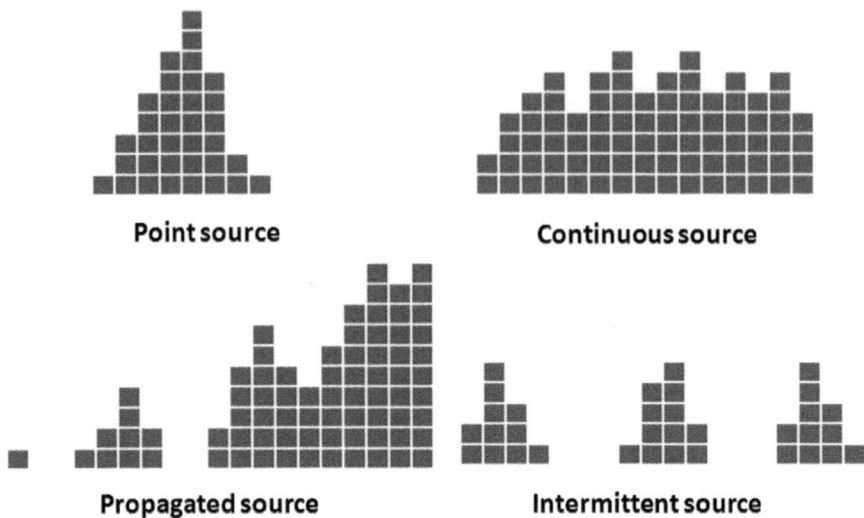

Fig. 15.1 Possible shapes of the epidemic curve. (Reproduced from: https://outbreaktools.ca/)

- In a *propagated outbreak* the curve will show an increase in cases after exposure, then fall in its number (after the exhaustion of those susceptible in the first exposure). Later a second increase happens (one incubation period after the peak of the first cases) due to secondary cases affected by cross-transmission.

Propagated source and continuous common source outbreaks are difficult to distinguish if just the curve shape is considered since the incubation period may be shorter than the rate at which cases decline after the initial exposure [19].

15.3.6.3 Spot Maps

A spot map gives a visual representation of the spread of the outbreak and may provide clues as to how the infection was transmitted. To draw a spot map, create a floor plan of the affected unit/ward. To show the relationship of the cases, mark them in the map as well as other potential reservoirs or sources of transmission (e.g. water sources, airflow, position of ventilation systems). In Fig. 15.2 it can be seen an example of a spot map of a geriatric ward of a Belgian hospital in which an outbreak of *Clostridium difficile* occurred in 2003 [20].

15.3.6.4 Gantt Chart

According to Last [2] the Gantt chart is a technique that graphically shows activities arranged by time and duration, but usually does not show interconnections among activities. In Fig. 15.3 it can be seen an example of this visualization technique of the same hospital outbreak referred in Table 15.4, in which each line refers to an identified case.

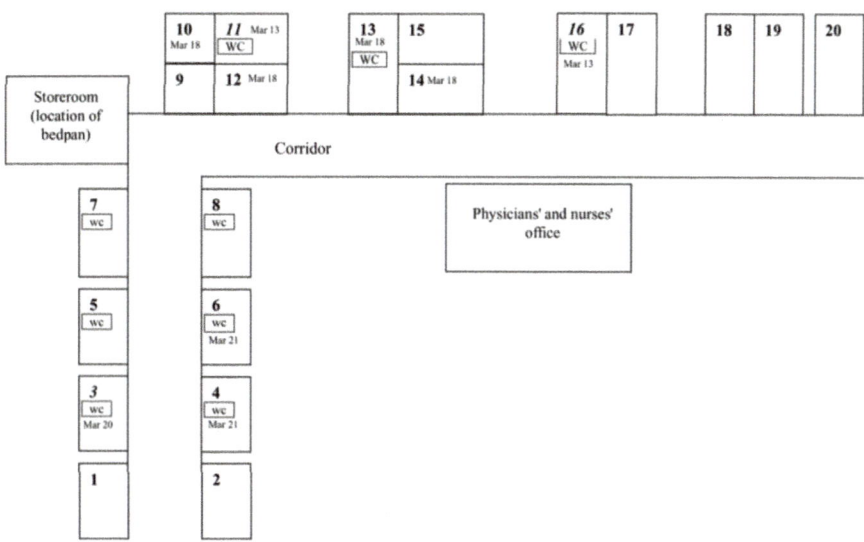

Fig. 15.2 Spot map of a geriatric ward of a Belgian hospital in which an outbreak of *Clostridium difficile*-associated disease occurred in 2003. Shown are the room numbers and dates on which cases were diagnosed. (Reproduced from Cherifi et al., 2006)

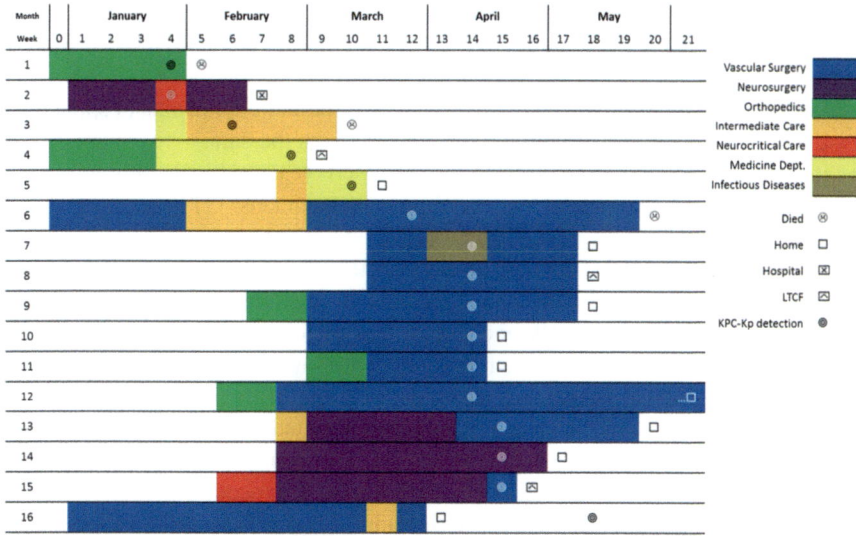

Fig. 15.3 Gantt chart applied to a KPC-producing *Klebsiella pneumoniae* outbreak at a Portuguese university hospital. (Reproduced from Ref. [17])

Brady et al [21] evaluated infectious pathogen transmission data visualizations in outbreak publications. Among the data visualization types of the 30 papers analyzed, 10 (27%) were spot maps and 3 (8%) were Gantt charts.

Two concepts are important to address in this step: index case and attack rate.

- The *index or primary case* is the initial patient in the population of an epidemiological investigation. It may indicate the source of the disease, the possible spread and which reservoir holds the disease in-between outbreaks.
- According to Gordis [22], the *attack rate* is defined as number of people at risk in whom a certain illness develops divided by the total number of people at risk. The attack rate is useful for comparing the risk of disease in groups with different exposures and can be calculated specifically for a given exposure [23].

Many investigations, descriptive epidemiology is sufficient to determine the likely outbreak cause.

15.3.7 Develop and Evaluate Hypotheses

According to Last [2] a "hypothesis is a conjecture that can be tested and (potentially) refuted" and proposes a possible explanation for a phenomenon or event. This estimation is based on the information gathered and compiled in the previous step. The hypothesis must address the possible source, mode of transmission and exposure that resulted in the outbreak. For developing a hypothesis, the ICP should:

- Review the available data (based on the line list, epidemic curve and/ or spot map);
- Look for the patterns (or outliers) that emerge from the data;
- Review the available literature and talk to experts (e.g., public health, infectious disease physicians, hospital epidemiologists, statisticians) [1].

In many situations, the number of cases in the cluster is very small (less than five) or resources are insufficient to conduct analytical studies. In this cases a different approach (known as "quick and dirty") can be followed. In this strategy, the compiled information in the "descriptive epidemiology" is examined looking for patterns and hypothesis generated about the most probable sources and mode of transmission. Then, control measures are implemented directed to the probable source and mode of transmission identified. After implementing these measures, a surveillance period follows to detect additional cases (expecting that the outbreak has terminated). If this is not the case, either additional control measures are implemented, or it is decided to conduct epidemiologic studies to test the hypothesis [11].

Two types of analytic studies can be performed to test hypotheses: case–control or cohort studies. Each of these has advantages and disadvantages, which should be addressed before choosing one over the other (Table 15.5). A major consideration is whether the number of cases is sufficient to statistically identify the source and risk factors for that specific adverse event (characteristic called *statistical power of the study*). If

Table 15.5 Comparison between characteristics of cohort and case-control studies

	Cohort studies		Case-Control Studies
	Prospective	*Retrospective*	
A. Study group	Exposed persons: $(a + b)$	Exposed persons: $(a + b)$	Persons with the disease (cases): $(a + c)$
B. Comparison group	Nonexposed persons: $(c + d)$	Nonexposed persons: $(c + d)$	Persons without disease (controls): $(b + d)$
C. Outcome measurements	Incidence in the exposed $$\left(\frac{a}{a+b}\right)$$ and Incidence in the nonexposed $$\left(\frac{c}{c+d}\right)$$	Incidence in the exposed $$\left(\frac{a}{a+b}\right)$$ and Incidence in the nonexposed $$\left(\frac{c}{c+d}\right)$$	Proportion of cases exposed $$\left(\frac{a}{a+c}\right)$$ and Proportion of controls exposed $$\left(\frac{b}{b+d}\right)$$
D. Measures of risk	Absolute risk	Absolute risk	—
	Relative risk Odds ratio Attributable risk	Relative risk Odds ratio Attributable risk	— Odds ratio Attributable risk[a]
E. Temporal relationship between exposure and disease	Easy to establish	Sometimes hard to establish	Sometimes hard to establish
F. Multiple associations	Possible to study associations of an exposure with several diseases[b]	Possible to study associations of an exposure with several diseases[b]	Possible to study associations of a disease with several exposures or factors
G. Time required for the study	Generally long because of need to follow-up the subjects	May be short	Relatively short
H. Cost of study	Expensive	Generally less expensive than a prospective study	Relatively inexpensive
I. Population size needed	Relatively large	Relatively large	Relatively small
J. Potential bias	Assessment of outcome	Susceptible to bias both in assessment of exposure and assessment of outcome	Assessment of exposure
K. Best when	Exposure is rare Disease is frequent among exposed	Exposure is rare Disease is frequent among exposed	Disease is rare Exposure is frequent among persons with disease
L. Problems	Selection of nonexposed comparison group often difficult Changes over time in criteria and methods	Selection of nonexposed comparison group often difficult Changes over time in criteria and methods	Selection of appropriate controls often difficult Incomplete information on exposure

Reproduced from Ref. [22]

[a]Additional information must be available

[b]It is also possible to study multiple exposures when the study population is selected on the basis of a factor unrelated to the exposure

the number is too small, the study may not be able to identify the source or risk factor (*type II or beta error*) or erroneously identify them (*type I or alpha error*) [11].

The type of study to choose depends on several factors, such as the hypotheses to be tested, the frequency of the adverse event, the duration of the outbreak and, as already said above, the number of cases. Frequently it is necessary to conduct several studies (each testing one different hypotheses). Most of the data has already been collected for the cases in the previous steps. Now, the same data should be collected for the control subjects (in a case– control study) or the exposed non-case (in a cohort study), so that a specific risk factor can be assessed [11].

Table 15.6 describes a *Pseudomonas aeruginosa* outbreak in a Neonatal Intensive Care Unit in which a matched case-control study was conducted to identify risk factors for this microorganism. Kinsey et al [24] found that "after adjusting for gestational age, case patients were more likely to have been in a room without a point-of-use filter (odds ratio [OR], 37.55; 95% confidence interval [CI], 7.16–∞). Case patients had higher odds of exposure to peripherally inserted central catheters (OR, 7.20; 95% CI, 1.75–37.30) and invasive ventilation (OR, 5.79; 95% CI, 1.39–30.62)". Environmental study identified 67% of the 28 samples grew *P. aeruginosa*, indicating the source of outbreak was attributed to contaminated water.

Table 15.6 Results of the case-control study to investigate a *Pseudomonas aeruginosa* outbreak in a Neonatal Intensive Care Unit

Characteristics	Cases, No. (%) (N = 31)	Controls, No. (%) (N = 31)	Adjusted Exact OR	95% CI
Device exposure				
Naso or orogastric tube	30 (97)	25 (81)	5.53	0.60–270.4
Peripheral IV	21 (68)	19 (61)	1.54	0.46–5.36
Invasive ventilation	19 (61)	8 (26)	5.79	1.39–30.62[b]
Peripherally inserted central catheter	18 (58)	6 (19)	7.20	1.75–37.30[b]
Umbilical catheter	5 (16)	7 (22)	0.80	0.15–4.17
Eye exam	3 (10)	4 (13)	0.65	0.07–5.37
Medication/nutrition exposure				
Antibiotics[c]	28 (90)	20 (65)	1.35	0.35-5.19
Breast milk	28 (90)	26 (84)	1.52	0.22–12.11
Total parenteral nutrition	26 (84)	20 (65)	3.10	0.80–13.91
Lipids	19 (62)	18 (58)	1.39	0.42–4.69
Blood products	11 (35)	6 (19)	3.02	0.70–15.92
Formula	10 (33)	13 (43)	0.77	0.21–2.87
Maintenance fluids	10 (32)	12 (39)	0.80	0.20–3.17
Environment exposure				
Incubator	23 (75)	17 (54)	2.76	0.54–18.77
Humidity	12 (39)	9 (29)	1.87	0.47–7.91
Unfiltered water[d]	31 (100)	14 (45)	37.55	7.16–∞[b]

Reproduced from Bicking et al. (2017)
NOTE. *OR* odds ratio, *CI* confidence interval

15.3.8 Consider Environmental Assessment

According to the *Council for Outbreak Response: HAI and Antimicrobial-Resistant Pathogens* [10], "an environmental assessment is a systematic evaluation of environmental factors that may have contributed to an outbreak. The need for an environmental assessment is informed by epidemiologic and other findings from the investigation". As a daily activity in infection control, environmental assessments are performed to evaluate cleaning practices that include observations and interviews with staff. On the other hand, in an outbreak, the objective of the environmental assessment is to identify possible environmental risk factors implied in these adverse events, such as possible contaminated areas that permit contact between the disease agent and vulnerable persons or environmental conditions that allow microbial survival, growth and transmission [10].

It should be noted that *Centers for Disease Control and Prevention* (CDC) doesn't recommend "to conduct random, undirected microbiologic sampling of air, water, and environmental surfaces in health-care facilities" but to "conduct microbiologic sampling as part of an epidemiologic investigation or during assessment of hazardous environmental conditions to detect contamination and verify abatement of a hazard" [25]. Jarvis [11] reinforces this idea, when he says "environmental cultures should not be taken randomly, because many surfaces are contaminated with numerous microorganisms, perhaps including the microorganism being investigated. Positive culture results from such random sampling may be misleading, difficult to interpret, and often confusing to investigators". Another aspect to pay attention is that clinical laboratories usually don't perform environmental testing (nor are licensed to do this), so samples may need to be sent to a reference laboratory (10). An example where this environmental sampling was performed and supported the outbreak investigated, is the one referenced in Table 15.6.

15.3.9 Perform Infection Control Assessment and Implement Control Measures

The most important part of the investigation is the interpretation of the results gathered in the descriptive and analytic parts of the epidemiological investigation. In this interpretation of results, the *Bradford Hill Criteria* should not be forgotten [12].

Bradford Hill Criteria

A. Strength of association;
B. Consistency with other studies;
C. Temporality (exposure precedes effect),
D. Biologic plausibility,
E. Biologic (dose-response) gradient.

Before implementing specific measures, it is important to evaluate the implementation status of the major areas in infection prevention in that healthcare unit [13]. For this infection control assessment several tools are available, such as the CDC "Infection Control Assessment and Response (ICAR) Tool" [26] or the WHO "Infection Prevention and Control Assessment Framework at the Facility Level" (IPCAF) [27]. These distinct tools are structured in major infection control areas that are summarized in Table 15.7.

After you tested the hypotheses and did an infection control assessment, you should review and direct the infection control measures that were taken in Step 3. As said before, the investigation steps do not always follow this order and can happen simultaneously, based on the evolution of knowledge of the chain of infection that is causing the outbreak (infectious agent, reservoir, portal of exit, mode of transmission, portal of entry, and susceptible host). These control measures can be classified into three phases, namely:

- *Short term*: immediate, specific measures needed to stop the outbreak (eliminate, isolate or quarantine the source).
- *Medium term*: measures to prevent a future outbreak (transmission-based precautions, hand hygiene, etc.).
- *Long term*: measures to ensure and maintain a culture of safety (immunizations, education).

Published data refer that improvements in patient screening and surveillance are implemented 54% of the time, staff screening in 38% of outbreaks, isolation or cohorting in 32%, enhanced or revised sterilization or disinfection practices in 24%, modification of care or equipment in 23%, increased use of protective clothing in 19%, and ward closure in 11% [28]. These interventions are generally implemented

Table 15.7 Structure of the CDC and WHO infection control assessment tools

CDC "Infection Control Assessment and Response (ICAR) Tool" Modules	WHO "Infection Prevention and Control Assessment Framework at the Facility Level" (IPCAF) Core components
1. Training, Audits, Feedback	1. Infection Prevention and Control (IPC) program
2. Hand Hygiene	2. IPC guidelines
3. Transmission-Based Precautions	3. IPC education and training
4. Environmental Services	4. HAI surveillance
5. High-level Disinfection and Sterilization	5. Multimodal strategies for implementation of IPC interventions
6. Injection Safety	6. Monitoring/audit of IPC practices and feedback
7. Point of Care Blood Testing	7. Workload, staffing and bed occupancy
8. Wound Care	8. Built environment, materials and equipment for IPC at the facility level
9. Healthcare Laundry	
10. Antibiotic Stewardship	
11. Water Exposure	

Adapted from Refs. [26, 27]

simultaneously, in a multimodal and quality improvement strategy. Examples of infection control measures that can be implemented, include:

- About outbreaks in bronchoscopy, Culver et al state that "specific approaches (…) include formalized institutional monitoring of isolate patterns to detect trends early, predefined protocols for epidemiologic characterization of suspected outbreaks, and institution of quality control monitoring for all steps in instrument reprocessing [29],
- About environmental contamination in hospitals, Otter et al address interventions to reduce and contain the shedding of pathogens into the environment and interventions to improve the efficacy of cleaning and disinfection [30],
- About outbreaks linked to water-containing hospital equipment, Yiek et al state, among other measures, that staff "should be trained as well to raise awareness of the importance of proper handling and cleaning of such medical equipment". [31],
- About outbreaks in adult intensive care units, Al-Dorzi and Arabi conclude that "using antibiotics judiciously, addressing the outbreak source, and intensifying infection prevention best practices remain the most important interventions for outbreak prevention and control" [32].

Depending on the pathogenic agent, involvement of public health authorities and control measures extended to the community, or across healthcare units, may be needed. These control measures might include contact tracing, patient and staff screening and specialized environmental testing [13].

15.3.10 Maintain Surveillance and Communicate Findings

Continuous case finding and surveillance efforts, based on the refined case definition, should be maintained for some months after the outbreak to ensure it has ended [13].

Communication skills are needed during the outbreak and must be carefully planned and involving several parts, namely: the head and staff of affected units; hospital administration and management; patients; staff; public health authorities and the media [1]. Communication based only in emails is not considered sufficient and must be complement with meetings, where discussion is possible.

Regarding patients, Schaefer et al [33] recommends to:

1. Notify patients when they have experienced harm, including explaining how the harm or change to their health care status likely occurred;
2. Provide information patients need to identify and/or mitigate a potential harm, including available information regarding the breach or outbreak;
3. Notify patients when they have experienced an alteration in care that results from an outbreak or infection control breach.

Communication is also important after the outbreak. A detailed report describing it (including the investigation and control measures) should be written and based in the 10 investigation steps. In this document things that went well should be addressed: challenges and what needs to change. The purpose of this report is to document the investigation and management of the outbreak, allowing an opportunity for evaluation and reflection on the process. The main conclusions should be addressed in a final briefing involving the parts listed above. [1] Special attention to communication with the media is important, centralizing all information in one spokesperson (that should have, preferably, experience with media).

15.4 Conclusion

Outbreaks can occur in any healthcare setting and may involve a variety of pathogens and transmission vectors. An organized investigation using the steps outlined here (with epidemiological and laboratory diagnostic tools) will help the ICP to manage the outbreak. Several of the proposed interventions have been successful in containing outbreaks, considering as a launching point that basic infection prevention practices (such as hand hygiene, isolation precautions or adequate staffing ratios) are in place. It is important, too, to understand that prevention strategies need to be adapted according to the results of the investigation. To be successful in this process it is essential to have access to the necessary resources and to work as a team with the appropriate stakeholders. Adequate information and communication to all interested parts will avoid an unsafe environment for the patients and, simultaneously, protect those who care for them. This safety culture requires the commitment of all those involved (directors, stakeholders, professionals and patients) to contain and prevent future outbreaks.

References

1. WHO. Outbreak investigations in health facilities [online course]. World Health Organization; 2022. Available from: https://openwho.org/courses/IPC-outbreak
2. Last JM, editor. A dictionary of public health. New York: Oxford University Press; 2007.
3. Gregg M. Field epidemiology. New York: Oxford University Press; 2008.
4. Skwarecki B. Outbreak: 50 tales of epidemics that terrorized the world. Massachusetts: Adams Media; 2016.
5. Aspalter C, editor. COVID-19 pandemic—problems arising in health and social policy. Singapore: Springer; 2023.
6. WHO. WHO Director-General declares MPOX outbreak a public health emergency of international concern [internet]. World Health Organization; 2024. Available from: https://www.who.int/news/item/14-08-2024-who-director-general-declares-mpox-outbreak-a-public-health-emergency-of-international-concern
7. Hawker J, Begg N, Reintjes R, Ekdahl K, Edeghere O, van Stennfergen J. Communicable disease control and health protection handbook. 4th ed. Oxford: Wiley Blackwell; 2019.
8. ECDC. Core competencies for infection control and hospital hygiene professionals in the European Union. Stockholm: European Centre for Disease Prevention and Control; 2013.

9. WHO. Core competencies for infection prevention and control professionals. Geneva: World Health Organization; 2020.
10. CORHA. Chapter 5: Investigation & control. In: Principles and practices for healthcare outbreak response. 2nd ed. USA: The council for outbreak response: healthcare-associated infections and antimicrobial-resistant pathogens; 2024. Available from: https://www.corha.org/.
11. Jarvis WR. Investigation of outbreaks. In: Mayhall CG, editor. Hospital epidemiology and infection control. 4th ed. Philadelphia: Lippincott Williams & Wilkins; 2012.
12. King ME, Bensyl DM, Goodman RA, Rasmussen SA. Chapter 3: Conducting a field investigation. In: Rasmussen SA, Goodman RA, editors. The CDC field epidemiology manual. New York: Oxford University Press; 2019.
13. Christensen BE, Fagan RP. Chapter 13: Healthcare settings. In: Rasmussen SA, Goodman RA, editors. The CDC field epidemiology manual. New York: Oxford University Press; 2019.
14. CDC. Outbreak and case definitions [internet]. Centers for Disease Control and Prevention; 2024. Available from: https://www.cdc.gov/urdo/php/surveillance/outbreak-case-definitions.html
15. BMA. Staff screening and treatment after infection outbreaks—occupational health aspects [internet]. British Medical Association; 2019. Available from: https://www.bma.org.uk/media/1071/bma_staff_screening_and_treatment_after_infection_outbreaks_oct_2019.pdf
16. Haymann DL. Control of communicable diseases manual. 21st ed. New York: American Public Health Association; 2022.
17. Peres D, Figueiredo P, Andrade P, Rocha-Pereira N, Carvalho C, Ferraz R, et al. Outbreak of KPC-producing Klebsiella pneumoniae at a Portuguese university hospital: Epidemiological characterization and containment measures. Porto Biomed J. 2022;7(6):e186. https://doi.org/10.1097/j.pbj.0000000000000186.
18. WHO. Guidelines on prevention and control of hospital associated infections. New Delhi: World Health Organization, Regional Office for South-East Asia; 2002.
19. Dwyer DM, Groves C, Blythe D. Chapter 5: Outbreak epidemiology. In: Nelson KE, Williams CM, editors. Infectious disease epidemiology. 3rd ed. Jones & Bartlett Learning; 2014.
20. Cherifi S, Delmee M, Van Broeck J, Beyer I, Byl B, Mascart G. Management of an outbreak of Clostridium difficile-associated disease among geriatric patients. Infect Control Hosp Epidemiol. 2006;27(11):1200–5. https://doi.org/10.1086/507822.
21. Brady MB, VonVille HM, White JF, Martin EM, Raabe NJ, Slaughter JM, Snyder GM. Transmission visualizations of healthcare infection clusters: a scoping review. Antimicrob Steward Health Epidemiol. 2022;2(1):e92. https://doi.org/10.1017/ash.2022.237.
22. Gordis L. Epidemiology. 5th ed. Philadelphia: Elsevier Health Sciences; WB Saunders Co Ltd; 2013.
23. Chen Y, Aldridge T, Ferraro C, Khaw FM. COVID-19 outbreak rates and infection attack rates associated with the workplace: a descriptive epidemiological study. BMJ Open. 2022;12(7):e055643. https://doi.org/10.1136/bmjopen-2021-055643.
24. Bicking Kinsey C, Koirala S, Solomon B, Rosenberg J, Robinson BF, Neri A, et al. Pseudomonas aeruginosa outbreak in a neonatal intensive care unit attributed to hospital tap water. Infect Control Hosp Epidemiol. 2017;38(7):801–8. https://doi.org/10.1017/ice.2017.87.
25. Sehulster LM, Chinn RYW, Arduino MJ, Carpenter J, Donlan R, Ashford D, et al. Guidelines for environmental infection control in health-care facilities—Recommendations from CDC and the Healthcare Infection Control Practices Advisory Committee (HICPAC). Chicago: American Society for Healthcare Engineering/American Hospital Association; 2004.
26. CDC. Infection Control Assessment and Response (ICAR) tool for general infection prevention and control (IPC) across settings [Internet]. Centers for Disease Control and Prevention; 2024. Available from: https://www.cdc.gov/healthcare-associated-infections/php/toolkit/icar.html
27. WHO. Infection prevention and control assessment framework at the facility level [internet]. WHO; 2018. Available from: https://www.who.int/publications/i/item/WHO-HIS-SDS-2018.9
28. Sood G, Perl TM. Outbreaks in health care settings. Infect Dis Clin N Am. 2016;30(3):661–87. https://doi.org/10.1016/j.idc.2016.04.003.

29. Culver DA, Gordon SM, Mehta AC. Infection control in the bronchoscopy suite: a review of outbreaks and guidelines for prevention. Am J Respir Crit Care Med. 2003;167(8):1050–6. https://doi.org/10.1164/rccm.200208-797CC.
30. Otter JA, Yezli S, Salkeld JA, French GL. Evidence that contaminated surfaces contribute to the transmission of hospital pathogens and an overview of strategies to address contaminated surfaces in hospital settings. Am J Infect Control. 2013;41(Suppl 5):S6–11. https://doi.org/10.1016/j.ajic.2012.12.004.
31. Yiek WK, Coenen O, Nillesen M, van Ingen J, Bowles E, Tostmann A. Outbreaks of healthcare-associated infections linked to water-containing hospital equipment: a literature review. Antimicrob Resist Infect Control. 2021;10(1):77. https://doi.org/10.1186/s13756-021-00935-6.
32. Al-Dorzi HM, Arabi YM. Outbreaks in the adult ICUs. Curr Opin Infect Dis. 2017;30(4):432–9. https://doi.org/10.1097/QCO.0000000000000387.
33. Schaefer MK, Perkins KM, Link-Gelles R, Kallen AJ, Patel PR, Perz JF. Outbreaks and infection control breaches in health care settings: Considerations for patient notification. Am J Infect Control. 2020;48(6):718–24. https://doi.org/10.1016/j.ajic.2020.02.013.

Immunization and Vaccination Programs and Nurses Roles

16

Ber Oomen and Tihana Gašpert

16.1 Introduction

This chapter explores the crucial role nurses play in immunization and vaccination programs, emphasizing their importance in preventing disease outbreaks and maintaining community health. It highlights nurses' essential contributions in administering vaccines and educating the public. The chapter also examines the interprofessional collaboration among healthcare workers to enhance vaccination efforts. A detailed look at the European Union's health ecosystem showcases key vaccination platforms and projects, such as the Coalition for Vaccination, and underscores industry partnerships in advancing vaccine development and distribution. Readers will gain an understanding of the multifaceted approach required to sustain effective immunization programs and improve public health outcomes.

Immunization and vaccination are vital public health practices that prevent infectious diseases by stimulating the immune system. They provide individual and community protection through herd immunity. The success of vaccination programs depends on public trust and acceptance, which healthcare professionals help foster. By examining the benefits of immunization and the need for high vaccination coverage, this chapter highlights the indispensable role of vaccines and nurses in safeguarding public health.

B. Oomen (✉)
European Specialist Nurses Organisation, Arnhem, Netherlands

T. Gašpert
University Hospital Rijeka, Rijeka, Croatia

Faculty of Health Sciences, University of Maribor, Maribor, Slovenia

16.2   Historical Context of Vaccination and Its Impact on Global Health

Vaccination is a form of infection prevention; by getting vaccinated, individuals protect themselves and contribute to public health by reducing the spread of infectious diseases [1]. However, the concept of vaccination did not emerge overnight. It was developed in response to past pandemics, progressing through trial and error, and led to today's advanced solutions. The development of vaccination was influenced not only by technical achievement but also by regional, national, and geopolitical factors, as well as budgetary and economic considerations [2].

Let's start with a one-liner on what is vaccination, "Vaccination is a form of infection prevention, by getting vaccinated, individuals protect themselves and contribute to public health by reducing the spread of infectious diseases[1]." But the whole concept of vaccination did not come with a straightforward line over processing, on the contra, it was a result of a response of great catastrophies from the past, finding a way out in pandemics causing havoc, by trial and error and towards today's innovative outcomes. This innovative process on development of vaccination was not only a process of technical achievement but also filled by periods of regional, national, and geographical political playfield and tensions. In this, we also see a special interplay between the public and private domain, with the public as the government and the civil society and the private with the industry. This whole evolution was also filled with cultural beliefs and processes of overcoming deep-rooted traditional assumptions and beliefs, even included the religion domain. And, as we are at the moment in this stage of innovation, there needs to be an acceptance that these dynamics will always be present and taken into serious consideration with new outbreaks, local, national, regional, or global.

The history of vaccination and its development is an impressive journey that has immensely shaped and impacted the public health. And in all this, we need to emphasize that all is first and primarily related to persons, taking risk and willing to go beyond the average in their motivation and dedication. The modern era of vaccination began in 1796 when Edward Jenner[2], developed the first successful smallpox vaccine using material from cowpox lesions. This groundbreaking discovery laid the early foundation for the development of vaccines but had still a long way ahead for acceptance. We also need to take in account the many professionals as the nursing professionals such as Isabel Zendal [3].

The twentieth century saw tremendous advancements in vaccine development. The introduction of the diphtheria, tetanus, and pertussis (DTP) vaccine in the 1940s, the polio vaccine in the 1950s, and the measles, mumps, and rubella (MMR) vaccine in the 1960s significantly reduced the incidence of these diseases worldwide. Smallpox, a devastating disease that claimed millions of lives, was declared

---

[1] https://www.who.int/news-room/questions-and-answers/item/vaccines-and-immunization-what-is-vaccination

[2] https://www.cdc.gov/smallpox/history/history.html

eradicated in 1980 following a global vaccination campaign led by the World Health Organization (WHO). This achievement remains one of the greatest triumphs in public health history.

The impact of vaccination on global health cannot be overstated. Vaccines have saved millions of lives, prevented countless cases of disease, and contributed to the near-eradication of several infectious diseases. For instance, polio, once a major cause of paralysis and death, has been eliminated from most parts of the world, with ongoing efforts to achieve complete eradication. Similarly, widespread vaccination has led to a dramatic decline in the incidence of measles, rubella, and whooping cough. This achievement marks a significant distinction from the pre-vaccination era when infections were the leading cause of death.

In all of this, it's important to recognize that new emerging infectious diseases frequently arise, driven by regions reluctant to vaccination, with significant social impacts, especially on children, young people, and early adults.

But we also need to emphasize that new outbreaks are constantly on the lure, especially when health systems collapse during regional conflicts and wars, as we saw in July 2024 during the war in Gaza with a Polio outbreak and dysentery and Hepatitis, triggered by a dysfunctional sewage and clean water supply and decrease of hygiene.

A major advancement in vaccine technology has been the use of messenger RNA (mRNA). Unlike traditional vaccines, which often use weakened viruses, mRNA vaccines introduce genetic material that instructs cells to produce a protein resembling that of the virus, triggering an immune response. This method allows for faster development, crucial in responding to rapidly spreading diseases. It also enables quick adaptation to new virus variants.

Because of the innovative aspect, the knowledge of health professionals at all levels, are well informed, share a unified message, each from their angle to strengthen trust in vaccines.

In conclusion, the historical context of vaccination highlights its profound impact on global health, underscoring the importance of continued investment in vaccine research, development, and distribution. The successes of the past provide a solid foundation for future efforts to prevent infectious diseases and improve public health outcomes worldwide.

16.3   Role of Healthcare Professionals in Vaccination

A crucial and often overlooked aspect in *sustainability of vaccination programs is the immense roles of professionals in the health domain*. And not only in the administration domain but also in policy and regulatory aspects—they all play an equally important role and share the responsibility. The success of vaccination depends not only on a well-functioning program and developed system but also on the personal motivation and dedication of professionals throughout the entire program chain. This includes developers, industry, clinical and operational professionals, as well as management, policymakers, and politicians. The success is ultimately based on the strength of the interconnected relationships between these groups.

The importance of *nurses and health professionals as advocates for vaccination* cannot be overstated, especially those in close contact with civil society and patients. As most of the communication are in the direct field between the professional delivering the vaccine and the receiver, the unique relation is also related that knowledge and experience are the drivers to overcome a negative attitude towards vaccination or hesitancy. History has shown how education, science, knowledge, and experience are the driving aspects overcoming obstacles and de-mystification. It deserved to underscore the nurses roles as they are for decades the most trusted professionals in the scope of the overall professionals, but it deserves a notification are at the same time, often the low or marginal in facilitation in time and finance in their continuing professional development and pathway.

It also deserves mention that collaboration with civil society organizations and patient organizations is essential to further elaborate on the role of professionals. Professionals cannot take the trust relationship for granted; it needs to be continuously reinforced, re-established, and maintained.

Often gaps in relations starts with small cracks at the top, and the dynamics need to be checked in an ongoing way, with a stable frequency. This is to gain trust on mutuality and equality. This also relates to the principle that all education and training materials should be consistent and accessible across all levels of complexity.

The absence of this creates a breeding ground for misinformation and leads to mystification. A fragile part is the misinformation in social media and only a harmonized and trustful message can overcome distrust.

While vaccination generally has the fewest adverse reactions and side effects compared to other medications, rare side effects are still reported.

It is of great importance that healthcare professionals are fully aware of this, as providing clear information to vaccine recipients is essential. In principle, every vaccine has potential side effects, and vaccination is inherently an intervention that may provoke such effects. By stimulating the immune system, vaccines elicit a natural response to help the body defend itself against invaders—this can be viewed as a positive outcome. However, negative side effects can occur when the vaccine triggers a chain of reactions that affect the patient's health, either in the short or long term. It is crucial that professionals are informed about these dynamics, know how to respond appropriately, and act with professionalism in their communication with national and international bodies when reporting these events.

16.4   Nurse Prescribing in Vaccination

Nurse prescribing refers to the official right granted to nurses to prescribe certain medications' [4] and on that domain, there is a rapid evolution in progress, although with great discrepancies in European context. While in some countries, nurses in specialist roles and those with advanced academic training have independent authorization to prescribe medication, in Eastern, Southern, and Mediterranean countries, there is a complete absence of such authority and autonomy.

Overall, there is much evidence that nurses are one of the best placed professionals in the vaccination domain, and the International Council of Nurses (ICN) has a clear position on this as stated in "The Role of Nurses in Immunisation, a snapshot from OECD countries" [5].

Interestingly, point number 4 in the overview of Key Findings Related to Nurses' Role in Immunisation in OECD Countries Surveyed states that "Prescribing is the largest barrier to nurses' increased involvement in immunisation." Regarding "Stakeholder Support" for nurse prescribing, it is noteworthy that, based on the data, the domain of physicians scored the lowest. This suggests that communication efforts should focus on identifying obstacles and exploring new directions to take.

Nurse prescribing in the global "immunization" is a powerful tool for preventing diseases and promoting health throughout life. Nurses play a crucial role in enhancing vaccination efforts by raising awareness about vaccines, dispelling fears, and educating patients and communities about the benefits of vaccination. With emerging roles for Advanced Practice Nurses (APNs) and Registered Nurses (RNs) in prescribing vaccines, they contribute directly to immunization efforts. Their involvement and expertise help increase vaccination rates and reduce vaccine hesitancy. By prescribing vaccines, nurses improve preventative health, reduce illness, and respond effectively to public health emergencies, thus enhancing community well-being.

16.5 Training and Continuing Education for Healthcare Professionals on Vaccination

Education and experience are the fundaments for quality and sustainability, and this has a specific status of professionals in health and with an emphasis on those fragile in health systems. Overall, education, training and professional development is, by history, the last post to invest. On the other hand, studies and data has shown that professionals feel rewarded and recognised when they are a part of the puzzle, a part of the solution, included in innovation, based on new knowledge and experience. Studies also have shown that nurses just arrived in clinics after basic graduation, they have not had any courses on vaccination, vaccinology, epidemiology, and microbiology. This contrasts with the fact that Florence Nightingale, the founder of the nursing profession, was highly prominent in both domains: infection prevention and the implementation of preventive measures.

In the second volume of this edition, the focus will first be on the importance of additional education for nurses during their early studies, as 'vaccination' is nearly absent from most nursing curricula. Additionally, post-graduation education, at the bachelor's and post-bachelor's career stages, will be emphasized, focusing on education, certification recognition, leadership, and mentoring. Most importantly, the goal is to create a standardized curriculum to ensure education is no longer ad-hoc and fragmented, lacking clear criteria and recognition of achievements.

16.6   Interprofessional Collaboration: Relation Between Health Professionals and Policy

The interprofessional collaboration involves administrators, educators, policymakers, and politicians working in concert. Their collective expertise ensures effective vaccine delivery, equitable access, and public health impact. As administrators, nurses are often the backbone of the healthcare system, yet they are frequently overlooked. They play a crucial role in the supply chain, provide essential advice on human resources, and foster communication among various healthcare disciplines to streamline the vaccination process.

Next, inter-collaborative and interdisciplinary education is crucial to ensure that everyone speaks with one voice and shares the same goals. This approach also contributes to safety and effective communication. Interprofessional education (IPE) equips professionals to work collaboratively across disciplines and fosters the cross-pollination of Continuing Professional Development (CPD) programs, such as those provided by the ECDC[3].

The other benefit is on policies and politics, as they are often interwoven. As policymakers are engaged in creating legislation and guidelines that shape vaccination programs, the process needs the support and endorsement of politicians, often in the position to allocate funding and address public concerns. In summary, interprofessional collaboration enriches the communication and provide positive impact on vaccination outcomes by leveraging expertise from various fields. By aligning administration, education, policies, and politics, we can achieve effective immunization strategies that benefit all.

16.7   Interprofessional Context in Vaccination Programs

There is significant variation in the role of nurses related to medication, and this is also reflected in their involvement in vaccination programs, including leadership, prescribing, and administration. The publication by Tinne Dillens and Eveline de Baetselier, *Perspectives of Nurses' Role in Interprofessional Pharmaceutical Care across 14 European Countries: A Qualitative Study in Pharmacists, Physicians, and Nurses* [6], highlights this uncertainty. This uncertainty and fragmentation create instability in the European contextual approach. While some countries have very successful interprofessional vaccination initiatives, in others, it's unimaginable for nurses to play a role. This is a flagrant observation, as Europe is a relatively small continent with many countries, each having its own policies. This leads to the conclusion that strategies are needed to foster interprofessional education, training, teamwork, and collaboration.

---

[3] https://www.ecdc.europa.eu/en/training/professional-development

16.8 Vaccination Platforms and Projects in the EU Health Ecosystem

This section provides an indication on the spectrum of many European initiatives related to vaccination, including European institutions, NGO (Nongovernmental Organization), alliances, and platforms. Throughout these efforts, the main driving force is ensuring consistency in information and uniformity in messaging, especially because vaccination is sensitive to misinformation and myths. For nurses, it is crucial to participate at all levels of policy, programs, and advisory roles.

- Institutional
  - European Commission
    EUVABECO, funded by the European Commission's EU4Health program—a project that aims to equip European Union Member States with validated implementation plans for innovative vaccination strategies and tools;
  - EMA
    LINK predominantly relates to COVID-19
  - ECDC
    LINK Immunisations and Vaccines
    ECDC training in the area of vaccination and vaccine hesitancy for primary healthcare professionals
    https://vxtrain.aspher.org/
    is funded by the European Centre for Disease Prevention and Control via Framework Contract ECDC/2021/005.
  - EU Joined Action on vaccination
    LINK ended program with Specialist Nurses as Stakeholder
  - WHO: #VaccinesWork campaign
  - European Unions Vaccination Portal
    European Vaccination Information Portal https://vaccination-info.europa.eu/en

Non-governmental Organizations (NGO)

- Coalition on Vaccination: Immunion
  Improving the uptake of vaccines across Europe. The Coalition for Vaccination works to deliver better vaccine education to healthcare professionals and better information to the general public.
  https://coalitionforvaccination.com/
- ESWI
  Our mission is to reduce the burden of major acute respiratory virus infections by fostering stakeholder communication and cross-disciplinary research in Europe.
  https://www.eswi.org/
- Coalition for Life-Course Immunisation (CLCI)

The Coalition for Life-Course Immunisation (CLCI) is a vibrant European network of experts, public health advocates, academics, and healthcare professionals. Our commitment is to prevent infectious diseases throughout all stages of life by promoting the benefits of broad-scale immunization.

https://www.cl-ci.org/

- Vaccine Safety Initiative (VIVI)

  The Vaccine Safety Initiative (VIVI) is an international scientific think tank and non-profit research organization. It is our mission to promote science-informed infectious diseases and vaccine safety research and communication; To stimulate thinking around key concepts and drive innovation in a globalized healthcare setting; To facilitate the implementation of high standards in vaccine safety and efficacy; To provide a platform for international and interdisciplinary scientific collaboration in infectious diseases and vaccines.

  https://www.vi-vi.org/

- European Patient Forum

  The European Patient Forum has a special policy related to vaccination and is actively campaigning on the field of vaccination to the civil society and its members.

  https://www.eu-patient.eu/policy/Policy/vaccination/

- Steering Group Influenza

  Seasonal influenza poses a significant but often under-recognized challenge to national health systems across Europe. Despite influenza vaccines being available for decades, influenza still has one of the highest and recurring impacts in terms of incidence and mortality among vaccine-preventable diseases and is estimated to cause up to 70,000 deaths in the EU each year, particularly among older adults and other at-risk groups.

  https://www.vaccineseurope.eu/

Private-oriented organization

- Vaccines Today platform

  Vaccines Today is an online platform focused on vaccination. Its target audience is the general public and others in Europe with an interest in immunization. The initiative is supported by Vaccines Europe—a trade association for vaccine manufacturers. Vaccines Today is a member of the WHO's Vaccine Safety Net network of trusted immunization websites Vaccines Today

16.9 Vaccines Industry's Role and Nurses Relation

The pharmaceutical industry plays a crucial role in developing, producing, and distributing vaccines, investing heavily in research and development to create effective solutions against various diseases. They operate within strict regulatory frameworks to ensure the safety and efficacy of vaccines, which involves conducting clinical trials and collaborating with health organizations. Specialist nurses are vital in this process as they administer vaccines and educate patients about their benefits and potential side effects. Acting as the primary point of contact during vaccination, nurses use their expertise to assess patient needs, manage vaccine storage, and maintain accurate vaccination records.

Despite their critical role, nurses often perceive themselves as distanced from the pharmaceutical industry, primarily because their focus is on patient care rather than the commercial aspects of healthcare. This perceived distance can stem from ethical concerns about the profit motives of the pharmaceutical industry or a lack of direct involvement in the development of vaccines. However, nurses are integral to the pharmaceutical ecosystem. Their collaboration with the industry is essential for successful vaccine rollouts, with their feedback on administration and patient reactions informing future vaccine development and policy decisions.

Moreover, continuous education provided by the pharmaceutical industry helps nurses stay updated on the latest advancements, ensuring that patients receive the best care based on current research. Thus, while nurses may feel distanced from the industry's commercial side, their role in patient care makes them indispensable to the effective deployment of vaccines. Recognizing this integrated relationship can enhance collaboration and improve public health outcomes.

16.10 Conclusion

In conclusion, immunization and vaccination programs represent a cornerstone of global public health, and nurses play an indispensable role in ensuring their success. Through direct patient care, public education, and interprofessional collaboration, nurses contribute to improving vaccination uptake, reducing vaccine hesitancy, and fostering trust in healthcare systems. As frontline healthcare workers, their involvement extends beyond administration to include advocacy, leadership, and, where allowed, prescribing roles, further empowering them to influence public health positively. Continuous professional development and collaboration with industry and policymakers are critical for equipping nurses with the necessary skills and knowledge to navigate the evolving landscape of vaccination. By strengthening these partnerships, nurses will continue to be pivotal in combating infectious diseases and advancing global health security.

References

1. Riedel S. Edward Jenner and the history of smallpox and vaccination. Proc (Bayl Univ Med Cent). 2005;18(1):21–5. https://doi.org/10.1080/08998280.2005.11928028.
2. Orenstein WA, Offit PA, Edwards KM, Plotkin SA. Plotkin's vaccines. 7th ed. Philadelphia: Elsevier; 2017.
3. Hatfield P. Isabel Zendal: the history of a Spanish nurse and her humanitarian work during the smallpox pandemic. La Marquesita Books; 2022.

4. Maier CB. Nurse prescribing of medicines in 13 European countries. Hum Resour Health. 2019;17(1):95. https://doi.org/10.1186/s12960-019-0429-6.
5. International Council of Nurses (ICN). Immunisation: nurses on the front line [Internet]. Geneva: ICN; 2017. [cited 2024 Oct 4]. Available from https://www.icn.ch/sites/default/files/inline-files/IMMUNISATION_Report%20%28002%29.pdf
6. De Baetselier E, Dilles T, Batalha LM, Dijkstra NE, Fernandes MI, Filov I, Friedrichs J, Grondahl VA, Heczkova J, Helgesen AK, Jordan S, Keeley S, Klatt T, Kolovos P, Kulirova V, Ličen S, Lillo-Crespo M, Malara A, Padysakova H, Prosen M, Pusztai D, Riquelme-Galindo J, Rottkova J, Sino CG, Talarico F, Tziaferi S, Van Rompaey B. Perspectives of nurses' role in interprofessional pharmaceutical care across 14 European countries: a qualitative study in pharmacists, physicians and nurses. PLoS One. 2021;16(5):e0251982. https://doi.org/10.1371/journal.pone.0251982. PMID: 34043650; PMCID: PMC8158867

Nurse Curriculum

17

Ber Oomen and Tihana Gašpert

17.1 Introduction

Infection prevention and vaccination are critical components of modern healthcare, yet the role of nursing in these areas often lacks standardization. Nurses, as key healthcare providers in health systems, playing an increasing role in vaccination administration, but also in program management, patient education, interprofessional education and in the overall infection control. However, disparities in education, training, certification, and educational standards across the European regions lead to inconsistent competencies and care outcomes [1, 2]. The absence of a unified framework limits the competencies of nurses to fully exercise their professional autonomy and expertise in this field and also leaves a missed opportunity in the full European vaccination program.

This chapter aims to propose a standardized postgraduate complementary curriculum for nurses, focused specifically on vaccination. Such a complementary curriculum would serve as a cornerstone for continuing professional development, ensuring that nurses not only maintain their skills but also grow as leaders in public health and advocate on vaccination. By establishing clear educational pathways and certification standards, this initiative seeks to harmonize nursing education across European borders, ensuring that all nurses, regardless of location, are equipped to meet the challenges of infection prevention.

The core objective of this proposal is to highlight how standardized education can enhance professional autonomy for nurses. Through a fundamental and well-structured curriculum, nurses would gain advanced competencies in vaccination,

B. Oomen (✉)
European Specialist Nurses Organisation, Arnhem, Netherlands

T. Gašpert
University Hospital Rijeka, Rijeka, Croatia

Faculty of Health Sciences, University of Maribor, Maribor, Slovenia

© The Author(s), under exclusive license to Springer Nature Switzerland AG 2025
B. Oomen, S. Gastaldi (eds.), *Principles of Nursing Infection Prevention Control*,
Principles of Specialty Nursing, https://doi.org/10.1007/978-3-031-84469-0_17

reinforcing their leadership roles in healthcare. This standardization would also ensure uniformity in care delivery, reduce fragmentation in nursing education, and promote a national framework that aligns with global best practices. Ultimately, this initiative will empower nurses to take greater responsibility and their accountability in vaccination and ultimately contribute significantly to infection prevention efforts.

With the right positioning on education and training, nurses possess the knowledge to address common myths and concerns with accuracy and empathy. Their close, ongoing relationships with patients and civil society make them best approachable, allowing them to provide credible, evidence-based information in a professional, personal way.

When well placed in crucial roles, nurses can lead public health efforts to counter misinformation, acting as trusted advocates for science and health literacy. Their ability to blend medical expertise with strong communication skills makes them uniquely to bridge between healthcare providers and the public, ensuring that accurate information reaches those who need it most. Empowering nurses to lead in this area not only enhances public trust but also plays a critical role in improving vaccination uptake and combating the spread of misinformation that threatens public health.

17.2   Redefining the Role of Nurses in Vaccination: A Paradigm Shift

For many years, the administration of vaccinations has been seen primarily as a responsibility belonging to the medical domain, with nurses playing a supportive role, this given the fact that expert platforms are mainly led by professionals in the medical domain. This traditional assumption, however, fails to recognize the evolving expertise and critical contributions that nurses make in the broader spectrum of healthcare, especially in vaccination programs. As healthcare systems face growing complexity and increasing demands for efficiency, it is essential to challenge this outdated perspective.

A paradigm shift is needed—one that acknowledges nurses not only as vaccinators but also as key stakeholders in vaccine education, strategy development, and public health advocacy. Nurses possess the clinical knowledge, patient rapport, and community trust necessary to lead vaccination efforts effectively. Their proximity to patients and families makes them invaluable in addressing concerns, dispelling myths, and increasing vaccine acceptance. Empowering nurses to take ownership of this critical role will lead to more integrated and holistic vaccination programs.

However, this shift requires more than just policy changes—it demands open and honest conversations across all levels of healthcare. Medical professionals, policymakers, and nursing leaders must engage in dialogue to address concerns, share insights, and build a consensus on the expanding role of nurses in vaccination. Through these discussions, we can foster a collective approach where all voices are heard, and the ultimate wisdom emerges not from a single profession but from interdisciplinary collaboration.

Embracing this change also requires bravery. Nurses, healthcare leaders, and policy-makers must openly challenge the status quo, advocating for expanded nurse autonomy and recognition of their competence in vaccination. It is time to move beyond the entrenched view that vaccination is solely a medical responsibility, and instead promote an inclusive approach where nurses play a leading role. In this collective effort, the shared wisdom and experience of all stakeholders will drive the success of future vaccination programs, creating a more resilient and unified healthcare system.

17.3 The Need for Standardization in Nursing Competencies

The lack of a standardized approach to education and certification in nursing creates significant disparities in competencies, practice, and expectations. In many European regions, nursing education related to infection prevention and vaccination is highly inconsistent, with each nation and even institutes or local authority implementing its own guidelines. This also on position and autonomy. In some European nations, nurses have a central role in the overall management, while in other regions, nurse positions are marginalized. This fragmented approach leads to uneven skill levels, varied knowledge bases, and differing clinical practices among nurses, which ultimately affects the quality of care delivered but also the preparedness of nurses and their motivation. Nurses may face uncertainty regarding their roles and responsibilities in vaccination efforts, leading to confusion and missed opportunities for professional growth. The overall absence also impacts their personal and professional self-esteem.

Inconsistent education has a direct impact on vaccination outcomes but also uptake what has a significant impact with overall declining uptakes across the European continent [3]. When nurses are not uniformly educated and trained, their ability and competencies to deliver vaccinations safely, provide consistent literacy and communication effectively, and confidently can vary. This variability can lead to errors in vaccine administration, patient hesitation, or inadequate infection control measures. Patients may receive mixed messages about vaccine safety or efficacy, further complicating public health efforts. A lack of standardized competencies among nurses compromises not only individual patient care but also community health outcomes [4].

A European standardized curriculum for nurses in vaccination is essential to address these inconsistencies. By aligning education and certification across the countries and in European context, a framework would ensure that all nurses, regardless of their European geographical location, possess the same level of expertise and are held to the same expectations. This would improve patient outcomes, enhance public trust, and support a more cohesive, efficient healthcare system but above all, the overall uptake of nurses themselves and the civil society. Moreover, a unified curriculum would empower nurses with the autonomy to take on greater leadership in infection prevention and vaccination initiatives but also interprofessional communication and uniformity in narratives. This is also needed to avoid further confusion in the campaigning on vaccination in relation to misinformation.

Certification is a vital tool for both professional development and competency assurance. A formal certification process linked to the curriculum would validate nurses' skills and knowledge in vaccination and infection prevention. This credential would not only recognize their expertise but also provide a pathway for career advancement, increasing job satisfaction and professional standing. Moreover, certification ensures a measurable standard of competency across the profession, fostering public trust in nurses as vaccine administrators and infection prevention leaders.

17.4 Nursing Expertise and Autonomy in Practice

For nurses to assume leadership roles in vaccination and infection prevention, they must possess a core set of competencies that performs basic clinical competencies. This a challenging issue as microbiology, infection prevention and vaccinology has a low status in the education programs. These competencies need to include a deeper understanding of immunology, vaccine pharmacology, and program management. In addition, nurses must be adept at patient education, able to communicate complex medical information clearly and empathetically. Leadership in this domain also requires strong decision-making abilities, critical thinking, and the capability to collaborate in multidisciplinary teams. With these competencies, nurses can take on expanded roles as public health advocates and key decision-makers in vaccination strategies.

Standardization in nursing education plays a crucial role in enhancing nurses' ability to make autonomous decisions. By equipping nurses with uniform, evidence-based knowledge and skills, a standardized curriculum empowers them to assess clinical situations independently and make informed decisions in vaccination administration. This not only improves the efficiency and accuracy of vaccine delivery but also enhances public health outcomes and the expected uptake rates. With a strong foundation in vaccination programs, nurses can confidently implement immunization initiatives, address patient concerns effectively, and respond to emerging health threats with minimal reliance on external guidance.

While structured education provides a framework for consistency, it does not stifle innovation or flexibility in nursing practice. On the contrary, standardization fosters autonomy by ensuring that nurses have the knowledge and confidence to operate independently. With clear guidelines and competencies in place, nurses are better equipped to adapt to local health needs, innovate within their roles, and take initiative in developing tailored vaccination strategies, thus balancing the need for standardization with the freedom to exercise professional judgment.

For education materials, there is an overall abundance of publications throughout nursing institutes and also in European context, such as the publication of the Nurses

Information and Communication Guide on Vaccination. These publications are highly valuable and are efforts towards a standardization of information,

17.5 Designing a Postgraduate Nurse Curriculum for Vaccination

A standardized nurse curriculum for vaccination should include key topics essential to developing comprehensive expertise. *Immunology* forms the foundation, helping nurses understand how vaccines interact with the immune system. Detailed instruction on *vaccination schedules* is critical, covering age-specific guidelines, contraindications, and the importance of timely immunizations. *Patient communication* is another essential component, focusing on how to effectively address vaccine hesitancy, provide clear information about benefits and risks, and build patient trust. Training in *adverse event management* is equally important, equipping nurses with the knowledge to recognize, respond to, and report potential side effects, ensuring patient safety and confidence.

To ensure the nationwide adoption of this curriculum, careful consideration must be given to European, national, regional, and institutional differences. A *flexible, modular approach* allows institutions to tailor the curriculum to local needs without sacrificing core competencies. *Stakeholder collaboration* with nursing schools, healthcare organizations, and regulatory bodies is key to ensuring buy-in and alignment with national health objectives. *Ongoing professional development and substantial facilitated programs* will be needed to ensure that the European nurses in all specialties and health domains remain current with evolving best practices in vaccination and infection prevention, further enhancing the curriculum's long-term effectiveness.

17.6 Conclusion and Future Directions

Standardizing a vaccination curriculum for nurses is crucial to ensuring consistent, high-quality care in infection prevention. A unified curriculum not only strengthens the knowledge and competencies of nurses but also enhances their leadership role in public health initiatives [5]. By providing clear guidelines on key areas such as immunology, vaccination schedules, and patient communication, a standardized approach ensures that nurses across regions deliver consistent and effective care, improving vaccination outcomes and public trust.

The advantages of a standardized vaccination curriculum are wide-reaching.

- **Improved care quality** is a key outcome, as nurses are uniformly equipped with the necessary skills to administer vaccines safely and confidently.
- **Reduced education fragmentation** in minimizes disparities in practice, ensuring that all nurses, regardless of location, meet the same competency standards.

- *Enhanced nursing leadership*, empowering nurses to take greater responsibility in vaccination efforts and infection prevention, ultimately contributing to better public health outcomes.

To implement this curriculum, *stakeholder engagement* is vital, with a proactive attitude from all domains and in a shared responsibility. Collaboration with nursing associations, educational institutions, and healthcare policy-makers will ensure that the curriculum aligns with national health goals and regional needs. *Policy advocacy* will also be necessary to push for curriculum adoption at the national level, emphasizing the importance of certification and continuing professional development. Potential challenges, such as resistance to change and regional disparities in resources, must be addressed with flexible implementation strategies and ongoing support for institutions and educators.

References

1. Nurses ICo. Nurses: a voice to lead a vision for future healthcare. Pon J Nurs. 2021;14(2):25.
2. Wakefield M, Williams DR, Le Menestrel S. The future of nursing 2020–2030: charting a path to achieve health equity. Washington, DC: National Academy of Sciences; 2021.
3. Lip A, Pateman M, Fullerton M, Chen H, Bailey L, Houle S, et al. Vaccine hesitancy educational tools for healthcare providers and trainees: a scoping review. Vaccine. 2023;41(1):23–35.
4. Tønnessen S, Scott A, Nortvedt P. Safe and competent nursing care: an argument for a minimum standard? Nurs Ethics. 2020;27(6):1396–407.
5. Stievano A, Caruso R, Friganović A. The specialist nurse in European healthcare 2030: ESNO congress 2024 highlights. Healthcare. 2024;12(16):48. MDPI

IPC and Holistic Approaches

18

Maria Mongardi

18.1 Introduction

Infection prevention and control (IPC) interventions are essential for the management of healthcare-associated infections (HAIs) and antimicrobial stewardship to ensure patient safety. Practicing prevention leads to lower HAI incidence and reduced antimicrobial prescriptions—an evident fact. Healthcare organizations have "care" embedded in their DNA, which partly explains the challenges in implementing preventive interventions across various care settings. Healthcare workers currently engaged in residential elderly care facilities, home care, and community hospitals have typically developed their professional backgrounds within hospital-based systems, carrying with them a hospital-centered cultural paradigm. Training and time are required to shift and adapt this paradigm to new care contexts.

International literature from the past decade highlights numerous determinants influencing IPC, including the culture of professionals, top management, healthcare organizations, patients, caregivers, and citizens. Other determinants include the organizational structure of care, staffing levels and composition, workplace climate, professionals' lifelong learning, interprofessional collaboration, as well as available financial resources, the presence of Infection Preventionists (IPs), and structural and material resources. This extensive list, with each factor holding equal importance and impact, illustrates a system complexity that inevitably calls for a paradigm shift.

IPC demands a holistic approach; without it, interventions will be insufficiently effective and efficient. The term "holistic" is derived from the Greek word "holos," meaning "whole," "totality," or "completeness." The adjective "holistic" refers to an approach or theory that considers the entire system rather than individual parts, implying the examination of the system as a whole and its complex

M. Mongardi (✉)
University of Parma, Emilia-Romagna, Italy

Scientific Society of Infection Risk Specialist Nurses (ANIPIO), Bologna, Italy relationships—an essential perspective for effective comprehension. We speak of holistic medicine, holistic science, holistic business management as opposed to traditional management, and a holistic approach to sustainable development. Today, a holistic approach to IPC is necessary both in concept and in action.

Holism emerged in the West in the 1920s, though the holistic approach in medicine dates back to Ancient Greece during the time of Hippocrates (450–350 BCE), making this idea far from new.

Governance of the holistic approach to IPC, within the complexity of healthcare organizations, requires what Edgar Morin's Complexity Theory describes as "well-made heads," meaning skills and competencies in management, leadership, strategy, communication, interpersonal relations, and information, in addition to specialized knowledge and skills in infection risk management.

18.2   IPC Culture

Culture is often regarded as the "software" that individuals use in their daily lives; it is commonly described as an inherent set of assumptions, values, and basic norms. Numerous theoretical and practical debates and discussions exist on the concept of culture. The various ways people think, feel, and act reveal cultural perspectives, and as such, culture should be considered in plural—as "cultures."

Cultural sensitivity, understood as the ability to enter and understand another's world, is not innate; it is learned through life experience.

IPC is contextually influenced, which necessitates a holistic approach beginning with a detailed analysis of enabling and hindering determinants, followed by planning strategic and priority interventions accordingly. Integrating a new set of evidence-based practices (EBP) in infection control into a culture is challenging, especially when these practices align with the core of the existing culture; if they do not, the challenge can be even greater. IPC uses recognized effective tools, such as bundles for the prevention of specific HAIs, but their effectiveness is jeopardized if there is no culture of change and team spirit. Every day, all staff members must apply EBP in the care process to ensure bundle effectiveness. In this scenario, several factors come into play: the level of professional training, workplace well-being, workload, understaffing, care organization, and leadership, to name a few.

To act on or improve adherence to evidence-based practices, healthcare professionals need infection control management support and must experience a culture of safety within the healthcare organization. Management should systematically target objectives, allocate appropriate resources, and organize process implementation and control. Preventing HAIs (e.g., surgical site infections, urinary infections, pneumonia like HAP and VAP, *Clostridium difficile* infections) requires sound planning, management, control, intervention evaluation, and clear information and communication of results achieved through professional collaboration.

It is essential to acknowledge that change and improvement require effective leadership in addition to management; without these two elements, infection control activities are hindered. Leaders are central to any significant change effort. Without strong servant leadership, cultural changes either fail or do not begin at all. Charismatic leaders can inspire and gain followers—they speak to the heart, touching emotional and personal pride. According to Maslow's hierarchy, they address self-actualization and esteem needs.

The utility of international and/or national good practice guidelines and IPC implementation cannot be overlooked, but these must be adapted to the specific context of the country, region, healthcare organization, and operational unit. This adaptation process is complex and requires specialized competencies. Biomedical sciences need cross-pollination with human sciences to improve intervention effectiveness, along with interprofessional education for the development of an interprofessional identity.

In the field of infectious diseases, and beyond, culture influences citizens' health, and health literacy is a determinant of health. Here are a few examples of how culture shapes people's behavior toward infection risk. The first example is the influence of culture on HIV-related risk behaviors. Though with limited evidence, HIV prevention and intervention programs rooted in the culture of specific citizen groups tend to be more appealing, acceptable, and effective. A study underscores the need for greater clarity and transparency regarding how researchers conceptualize "cultural-based interventions" [1].

A second example involves a deeper understanding of conspiracy beliefs around COVID-19 vaccines. COVID-19 vaccination emerged as a key strategy to combat the global pandemic, and vaccine acceptance is an integral part of this process [2]. Studying the various factors influencing health behaviors and attitudes is crucial to effectively counter vaccine hesitancy.

Cultural rigidity is an important factor that influences human behavior and the way different societies address collective threats [3].

The third example concerns recurrent urogenital infections, such as bacterial vaginosis, vulvovaginal candidiasis, and urinary tract infections, which have high prevalence and significant psychosocial impact. A narrative review discusses the impact of common recurrent urogenital infections on psychosocial aspects, including quality of life, stress, mental health, sexual health, work productivity, and satisfaction with medical care. Education, awareness, and access to care can help alleviate the negative implications of recurrent urogenital infections [4].

Public culture regarding infection risk requires substantial investment. A study conducted in 1989 and repeated in 2019 interviewed 1004 U.S. consumers about their education and awareness of the risk and prevention of healthcare-associated infections (HAIs). Awareness of HAI risk remained stable (62% in 1989 vs. 65% in 2019), but the belief that HAIs are preventable decreased (from 83% to 28%). Healthcare professionals and the Internet remain the primary sources of information [5].

18.3   Patient Empowerment in Infection Prevention

In recent years, there has been growing interest in empowering patients to act as partners in healthcare-associated infection (HAI) prevention efforts and in the responsible use of antimicrobials. However, patients often have limited awareness of the risks of acquiring and spreading healthcare-associated pathogens and have received little information on how they could contribute to infection prevention efforts. Although patients are the primary focus of these initiatives, the inclusion of family members should be considered in many cases, as they often play an essential role in healthcare decision-making. While patient empowerment interventions may be beneficial on an individual basis, the long-term goal of these initiatives should be to define evidence-based educational "packages" implemented collectively to enhance patient engagement. One strategy for patient empowerment advocates could be to incorporate patients and families into educational packages of evidence-based practices (EBP) and patient safety initiatives.

Further research is necessary to determine effective ways to engage patients and to assess whether patient involvement can improve the implementation of evidence-based care packages. Patients could potentially participate in evidence-based efforts to reduce, for example, the overuse of antibiotics or prolonged use of urinary and central venous catheters and to improve healthcare staff hand hygiene. Beyond patient participation in developing EBP educational packages, it is necessary to establish aggregated measures that include other tools patients can use to reduce the risk of healthcare-associated infections. An integrated set of preventive measures may be more effective than single, focused initiatives, such as an educational package covering healthcare staff hand hygiene, patient hand hygiene, and surface sanitization. Simple measures, like enabling patients to monitor staff hand hygiene and promoting patients' personal hygiene, could prove beneficial. Another example of an educational package might involve Clostridium difficile patients, where a list of simple, common-sense measures could be useful to them and caregivers in avoiding cross-infections.

Empowering patients and their families as partners in infection prevention is a strategic intervention that requires a cultural shift. Education is critical for patient empowerment initiatives because patients are often unaware of the infection risk associated with medical and surgical procedures. Future objectives for patient empowerment could include: [1] the inclusion of patients and families in educational care packages, [2] the development of combined measures that all patients can use to reduce healthcare-associated infection risks, and [3] the creation of targeted combined interventions for patients infected by specific pathogens or specific populations with common risk factors (e.g., surgical patients).

Citizen empowerment is closely linked to health literacy, which is fundamental for empowerment. Health literacy encompasses the cognitive and social skills that determine individuals' motivation and ability to access, understand, and use information to promote and maintain good health. The development of cognitive and social skills also depends on exposure to different forms of communication and the content of messages based on the communication process (sender, medium,

Table 18.1 The three levels of health literacy by D. Nutbeam [6]

Domain	Abilities
Functional Health Literacy	Basic reading, writing, and literacy skills needed to understand health communications and use healthcare services. This level is not about decision-making but understanding instructions, with a passive patient role.
Interactive Health Literacy	A set of communication and social skills used to extract meanings from various forms of communication and apply new knowledge to changing circumstances, which increases personal independence but primarily benefits the individual.
Critical Health Literacy	The highest level of cognitive and social skills necessary for critically analyzing information and using it to exert greater control over life events and situations through individual and collective actions, addressing social, economic, and environmental determinants of health.

channel, signal, code, signal perception, receiver, decoding of the signal, and feedback).

Digital health literacy skills are also necessary to access, search, select, understand, evaluate, and apply health information available online or through digital applications. However, the gold standard would be to develop a health-literate healthcare organization, where top management integrates health literacy as an essential part of its mission, structure, and activities. This approach places the focus on people's competencies rather than system competencies.

D. Nutbeam's model [6] defines three levels of health literacy, each with corresponding abilities, as summarized in Table 18.1.

This framework enables individual and community empowerment.

18.4 Environmental Sustainability

Healthcare is one of the most important sectors in managing the effects of climate change and, at the same time, plays a significant role in reducing its own carbon emissions. Globally, healthcare is responsible for nearly 5% of total greenhouse gas emissions [7].

The HCWH Europe 2024–2029 manifesto [8] establishes ten policy priorities aimed at minimizing the environmental impact of healthcare, protecting and improving public health, urging pharmaceutical companies to reduce the negative environmental impacts of their products, and making healthcare systems eco-sustainable and future-ready. The ten policy priorities outlined in the HCWH manifesto are as follows:

1. Implement a One Health approach to antimicrobial resistance.
2. Set legally binding, more ambitious climate targets.
3. Integrate health into climate action.
4. Strengthen the climate resilience of healthcare systems.
5. Ensure a comprehensive chemical policy package that meets all commitments of the strategy for chemical sustainability.
6. Promote and enable circular economy practices within healthcare.

7. Build resilience and transparency in the healthcare supply chain.
8. Support the implementation of the United Nations General Assembly's 2024 targets on reducing antibiotic resistance.
9. Enforce corporate due diligence obligations.
10. Protect water quality for future generations.

This list reflects the cultural shift and commitment that healthcare organizations must undertake in relatively short timeframes. Requiring legally binding, more ambitious climate targets, integrating health into climate action, and strengthening the climate resilience of healthcare systems are major challenges. The healthcare sector, for instance, must take responsibility for the impact of its emissions on health and adopt measures to decarbonize in line with the Paris Agreement. Numerous actions can be implemented within a healthcare facility, starting with interventions to reduce the use of plastic, personal protective equipment, cleaning solutions, antiseptics, disinfectants, intravenous therapies, and single-use materials where reusable alternatives are available, and with better pharmaceutical management. Additionally, operational areas that deserve particular attention include operating rooms and units that care for especially vulnerable patients, such as neonatal and intensive care units, as well as practices that are more sustainable. Here are two examples: the first addresses making operating rooms more sustainable, and the second focuses on medication administration methods—some of which are more sustainable than others.

The environmental impact of surgical activities in operating rooms is high; thus, awareness and action to reduce this impact are essential without compromising care safety. In 2024, the National Federation of Orders of Surgeons and Dentists (OMCeO) of Turin and the Association of Physicians for the Environment (ISDE) Italy developed several information sheets, one of which outlines "How to make operating rooms more sustainable" and provides three practical actions: [1] Avoid preparing more sterile surgical kits than necessary; if their need for the procedure is uncertain, it is advisable to wait and open the kit during the procedure if required. Many sterilized surgical instruments are prepared and then not used. [2] Reduce water and energy consumption: after the first surgical handwashing with water and antiseptic of the day, alcohol-based hand rub can be used for subsequent procedures. [3] Prefer total intravenous anesthesia and aim to reduce or eliminate the use of desflurane and nitrous oxide. Additionally, there is overuse of single-use items in operating rooms, increasing waste without necessarily reducing infections. It is time to carefully evaluate which items must be single-use and which could be multi-use, prioritizing alternatives.

Another information sheet addresses medication administration methods, highlighting that "some routes of administration are more sustainable than others." In patient care, balancing therapeutic efficacy with environmental sustainability is increasingly important, as exemplified by medication use and administration choices. According to the WHO, the overuse of intravenous drugs, when oral formulations could be just as effective, is a significant global issue [9]. The three practical actions recommended by the OMCeO of Turin and ISDE Italy are: [1] Choose the oral route if the required dose is tolerable for the patient; oral formulations are commercially available, and there is no evidence supporting intravenous therapy use. [2] Switch from intravenous to oral therapy as soon as possible; current literature suggests that oral therapy is often as effective as continuing intravenous administration. [3] Provide education and training: healthcare professionals can contribute to changes prioritizing oral over intravenous drug use. We can promote a safer pharmacy that requires a shift in how we produce, use, and dispose of drugs.

From a circular healthcare perspective, the sector must limit unnecessary single-use products and chemicals and serve as an advocate for manufacturers. Therefore, reusable and nontoxic solutions that conserve natural resources, reduce waste, and are better for patients, economic impact, and the planet should be prioritized.

Purchasing and packaging should be closely monitored to make healthcare increasingly "Plastic Free," but this also requires political will, employee engagement, a review of care procedures, and much more. Health Care Without Harm (HCWH) Europe is an organization with the mission of creating a sustainable healthcare sector that does not harm patients or our planet. It has identified six categories of products on which work could reduce plastic use by up to 60%, including personal protective equipment, intravenous solutions, solution bags, syringes, diapers and incontinence materials, bed covers, and gloves [10].

A healthcare facility's mission is to preserve health, and thus sustainable healthcare is no longer a choice but a necessity. Climate-conscious healthcare is essential, as climate change contributes to the development of new infections and pandemics. Therefore, healthcare organizations must work to reduce their emissions. To achieve this, it is necessary to reevaluate IPC best practices, where single-use guidance plays a significant role.

18.5   Conclusion

Healthcare-associated infections (HAIs) present major challenges to healthcare systems, and surveillance of this phenomenon plays a crucial role in defining its scope. Traditional surveillance, although effective, is resource-intensive, and the development of new technologies, such as artificial intelligence (AI), can support traditional surveillance by analyzing an increasing volume of health data and meeting patient needs [11].

While digital tools show promise for HAI surveillance, particularly for surgical site infections (SSI), challenges remain in resource allocation and interdisciplinary integration within healthcare settings, highlighting the need for ongoing development and implementation strategies. The potential of AI to improve IPC is vast; however, AI alone will not enhance IPC. Sustainable improvements in IPC require a cultural and behavioral shift supported by appropriate governance structures.

Care safety policies, management skills, servant leadership, and adequate resources are the pillars for advancing IPC.

There is a growing interest in empowering patients as partners in infection prevention, with health literacy being essential, as patients are often unaware of infection risks [12]. This lack of awareness weakens their ability to prompt professionals to follow best prevention practices and national and local policies. Joint interventions are necessary to enhance patient empowerment.

One obstacle to IPC is the culture of healthcare professionals and organizations; changing this culture requires management strategies, humanistic competencies, on-the-job training, resources, and time. Another significant obstacle is the "historical DNA of hospital structures," which prioritizes care over prevention.

IPC must be renewed to align with eco-sustainable healthcare, reconsidering the use of single-use devices through careful evaluation of which items must be disposable and which can be reprocessed and reused. This challenge calls for new policies, cultural shifts, reengineering of certain processes, and procedural revisions.

These challenges must be addressed through a new team culture, leveraging the motivation of professionals, skill development, and fostering a team spirit centered on the value of care safety. Developing a culture of values can have a profound impact on care quality.

A holistic approach to IPC must consider all determinants that facilitate and hinder professionals' daily actions, the choices of top management, and the strategies to be implemented.

References

1. Vitsupakorn S, Pierce N, Ritchwood TD. Cultural interventions addressing disparities in the HIV prevention and treatment cascade among Black/African Americans: a scoping review. BMC Public Health. 2023;23(1):1748. https://doi.org/10.1186/s12889-023-16658-9. PMID: 37679765; PMCID: PMC10485990
2. Laine C, Cotton D, Moyer DV. COVID-19 vaccine: promoting vaccine acceptance. Ann Intern Med. 2020;174(2):252–3. https://doi.org/10.7326/m20-8008.
3. Gelfand MJ, Jackson JC, Pan X, Nau D, Pieper D, Denison E, et al. The relationship between cultural tightness-looseness and COVID-19 cases and deaths: a global analysis. Lancet Planet Health. 2021;5(3):e135–44. https://doi.org/10.1016/S2542-5196(20)30301-6.
4. Thomas-White K, Navarro P, Wever F, King L, Dillard LR, Krapf J. Psychosocial impact of recurrent urogenital infections: a review. Womens Health (Lond). 2023;19:17455057231216537. https://doi.org/10.1177/17455057231216537. PMID: 38099456; PMCID: PMC10725120
5. McGuckin M, Storr JA, Govednik J. Patient awareness of healthcare-associated infection risk and prevention: has there been a change in 3 decades (1989–2019)? Am J Infect Control. 2021;49(11):1448–9. https://doi.org/10.1016/j.ajic.2021.05.009.
6. Nutbeam D. Health literacy as a public health goal: a challenge for contemporary health education and communication strategies into the 21st century. Health Promot Int. 2000;15:259–67. https://doi.org/10.1093/heapro/15.3.259.
7. Watts N, et al. Report of The Lancet Countdown on health and climate change: responding to converging crises. Lancet. 2020;397(10269):129–70.
8. Health Care Without Harm (HCWH) Europe. For a sustainable healthcare system and healthier EU citizens: 10 policy priorities 2024–2029 [Internet]. Brussels: Health Care Without Harm (HCWH) Europe; 2023. Available from https://europe.noharm.org/resources/manifesto-sustainable-healthcare-system-and-healthier-eu-citizens
9. World Health Organization. The pursuit of responsible use of medicines: sharing and learning from country experiences. World Health Organization; 2012. Available at: https://iris.who.int/handle/10665/75828

10. Health Care Without Harm (HCWH) Europe. Measuring and reducing plastics in the health-care sector [Internet]. Brussels: Health Care Without Harm (HCWH) Europe; 2021. Available from: https://europe.noharm.org/sites/default/files/documents-files/6886/2021-09-23-measuring-and-reducing-plastics-in-the-healthcare-sector.pdf

11. Fitzpatrick F, Doherty A, Lacey G. Using artificial intelligence in infection prevention. Curr Treat Options Infect Dis. 2020;12(2):135–44. https://doi.org/10.1007/s40506-020-00216-7. Epub 2020 Mar 19. PMID: 32218708; PMCID: PMC7095094

12. Donskey CJ. Empowering patients to prevent healthcare-associated infections. Am J Infect Control. 2023;51(11S):A107–13. https://doi.org/10.1016/j.ajic.2023.03.008.